TESTIMONIALS

Bravo! Harvey Diamond has done it again. He clearly reveals how we can take charge of our own health and prevent disease.

— Dr. Wayne Dyer,
Author of *Manifest Your Destiny:*
The Nine Spiritual Principles for
Getting Everything You Want
and *Your Erroneous Zones*

Harvey Diamond gives everyone a powerful tool for the restoration of health. He speaks from a point of view so many of us now want: with an awareness of nature, consciousness and their role in healing. I deeply welcome this book into my own life.

— Marianne Williamson,
Author of *A Return to Love;*
A Woman's Worth; Illuminata

A magnificent job of ordering and documenting the vast body of information into a cogent, irrefutably sensible and wise program.

— Jesse Lynn Hanley, M.D.,
Director, Malibu Health and Rehabilitation

This is the health book we've been looking for. Harvey demystifies modern medicine's incurable disease, and puts you in charge.

— Marcus Laux, M.D.,
Editor, *Naturally Well*

This book represents the first ray of hope in conquering cancer. It could very well save your life or the life of someone you love.

— Dr. Gayle Black, Clinical Nutritionist,
President, Eating Smart Company

This book will empower as no medical encounter can with the knowledge and confidence to prevent disease naturally.

— Zoltan P. Rona, M.D.,
Columnist, *The Toronto S*

In my practice specializing in women's health, I have often wished for a book that would dispel the current hysteria and melodrama around disease. A book that would clearly and succinctly describe the changes necessary to prevent heart disease and cancer. A book that was engaging and easy to understand. A book that was free of preaching and dogmatic statements. A book that proposed simple changes that anyone could make no matter what the size of their pocketbook, or how difficult their circumstances. You hold such a book in your hands.

—Carolyn DeMarco, M.D.,
Author of *Take Charge of Your Body*

This extremely well-researched book sends a welcome message of hope to millions of potential victims.

—Edward A. Taub, M.D.,
Author of *Balance Your Body, Balance Your Life*

Harvey Diamond's belief that cancer is preventable goes along with my own experience, beliefs and research.

—Barbara L. Joseph, M.D.,
Author of *My Healing of Breast Cancer*

Mr. Diamond provides candid insight and powerful, beneficial advice for women in the challenge of the prevention of breast cancer.

—J. William La Valley, M.D.,
Founder, Complementary Medicine Section,
Canadian Medical Association

An empowering resource for anyone interested in improving the quality of their life, *Fit for Life: A New Beginning* delivers not only hope, but also the information you need to free yourself from fear.

—Anthony Robbins,
Author of *Awaken the Giant Within; Unlimited Power*

FIT FOR LIFE

A NEW BEGINNING

THE ULTIMATE DIET AND HEALTH PLAN

HARVEY DIAMOND

CITADEL PRESS
Kensington Publishing Corp.
www.kensingtonbooks.com

CITADEL PRESS BOOKS are published by

Kensington Publishing Corp.
119 West 40th Street
New York, NY 10018

All Kensington titles, imprints, and distributed lines are available at special quantity discounts for bulk purchases for sales promotions, premiums, fundraising, educational, or institutional use.

Special book excerpts or customized printings can also be created to fit specific needs. For details, write or phone the office of the Kensington sales manager: Kensington Publishing Corp., 119 West 40th Street, New York, NY 10018, attn: Sales Department; phone 1-800-221-2647.

ISBN-13: 978-0-8065-4117-4
ISBN-10: 0-8065-4117-2

First Kensington hardcover printing, May 2000
First Kesnington paperback printing (updated edition), January 2011
First Citadel trade paperback printing: March 2021

10 9 8 7 6 5 4 3

Printed in the United States of America

CONTENTS

EDUTRITION®

Definition: A blending of nutritional knowledge and educated application, with the aim of improved health and self-empowerment.

Perhaps the least explored area by the medical profession is the subject of nutrition. Yet proper nutrition is at the base of good health. As stated in a report written by Elizabeth Frazão in the USDA *Food Review* of 1996*: "Scientific evidence increasingly suggests that diet plays an important role in the onset of chronic diseases—contributing to increased illnesses, reduced quality of life, and premature death." To coin a phrase, "We are what we eat." A point I will continually make throughout this book is that diet—the seventy tons of food we eat during the course of our lives, along with the quantity and quality of fluids we consume—is the predominate determining factor in acquiring and maintaining vibrant health.

To that end I have chosen to use the term EDUTRITION®. My goal through the pages of this book is to *educate* you about *nutrition* and nutritional supplements, and how this information can empower you to make choices that will improve your health.

I will also introduce a number of experts in this book who will discuss a more recent phenomenon that is fast approaching epidemic proportions—autism, also known as autism spectrum disorders (ASD). These conditions have afflicted, according to the CDC in 2006, about one percent, or one child in every 110 [males: 1:70; females: 1:315]). The average prevalence of ASDs identified among children aged 8 years increased 57 percent in 10 sites from the 2002 to the 2006 ADDM surveillance year.* These are frightening statistics; even more frightening is the lack of EDUTRITION® in this area.

I will also supply you with information about where you can further your EDUTRITION®. These organizations and companies are in the forefront of nutrition and nutritional supplements, and also extremely knowledgeable in the area of ASDs. Please feel free to contact them for more information.

Nutritional Supplements

VP Nutrition
P.O. Box 188
Osprey, Fl 34229
Toll-free: 877-335-1509
Outside the United States: 941-966-9727
Website: www.vpnutrition.com

For updated information on this book

Website: www.fitforlifetime.com/links.php
VP Nutrition on Facebook
www.vpnutritionblog.com

FOREWORD

Fit for Life: A New Beginning is no ordinary book.

More than a review of diseases such as cancer or how to manage them, this important book makes the strategic transition from treatment to prevention. People are increasingly taking responsibility for decisions concerning their health. *Fit for Life: A New Beginning* empowers the individual to make health-care decisions that are based on personal research; indeed, it accelerates this process.

The traditional view of the doctor as all-knowing is undergoing dramatic change as people gain the knowledge to demystify medicine. What do physicians actually know about the cause of cancer, for example? Precious little. In fact, no one knows for sure what causes most cancer. And while heart disease is still the country's Number 1 killer, cancer is our greatest fear. Unfortunately, some cancers—breast cancer, for example—have been on the rise for decades. We still don't know why.

And so, back to Harvey Diamond and *Fit for Life: A New Beginning*. The book is not meant to be a medical textbook. Medical texts deal exclusively with diagnosis and treatment, while *Fit for Life: A New Beginning* covers a much broader landscape. While it does discuss diagnosis and treatment, its real message is that *you can prevent disease*. Moreover, where medical books are objective, analytical, and usually completely unexciting to read, this book is alive with real people, stimulating ideas, and commonsense approaches to how you can take control of your health. It beats with a heart of its own as it covers a number of areas: Natural Hygiene, inspiring recoveries, radical surgery, nutrition, the mind-body connection, vegetarianism, chemotherapy, exercise, radiation, the lymphatic system, and most important, the three principles of CAREing.

Fit for Life: A New Beginning is an exciting examination of a complex subject. Harvey Diamond penetrates much of its mystery with a prevention program couched in the life-sustaining principles of Natural Hygiene and an approach that challenges conventional thinking. He takes doctors to task for stubbornly clinging to the past for cancer diagnosis, management, and treatment. He discusses what, in his view, this disease is and proposes a simple, effective program to address its causes. But this isn't just somebody's theory or wild guess. Harvey Diamond's program is based on a growing body of sound scientific evidence from the world's most respected researchers. For example, he addresses the subject of women and breast cancer not only with passion, but with carefully compiled and analyzed facts and studies accrued from a number of reliable sources. He translates this information so that it is accessible to everyone, as only the author of the best-selling diet and health book of all time, *Fit for Life* (approximately 11 million copies in thirty-one languages), could do. He has also drawn from thirty years of his own study of diet and health, disease prevention, Natural Hygiene, yoga, and Eastern medicine.

Fit for Life: A New Beginning is enjoyable, inspiring, and will change how you live, eat, play, and think about disease. I know of no popular or scientific book on the subject that brings together the wealth of wisdom contained in these pages. Everyone should read it and reread it. It is a book with answers, a book of real hope. It will help end your fears about disease.

Harvey's program to promote and restore vibrant health allows you to enjoy that all-important sense of security you feel when you take responsibility for your own health. Once again you can feel renewed joy and hope knowing that a life free of the fear of disease such as cancer is an attainable goal.

I've treated thousands of cancer patients during my general surgery training. I participated in many radical cancer surgeries. These experiences were unpleasant, and the patients who endured these operations lost more than a breast, or stomach, or prostate. All too often the cancer would recur, and the hopelessness of a broken spirit would be added to a patient's physical plight. I had nothing more to offer medically, except morphine-type drugs when the pain became intolerable, and I felt each patient's despair. Occasionally I visited these patients in their homes. The fortunate ones had loving families and supportive religious beliefs that saw them through. I felt strongly that we in medicine had to find a way to stop this awful disease that destroyed so many lives. I knew, however, that there was very little we could do. Until now. Until *Fit for Life: A New Beginning*. What makes me excited about Harvey Diamond's program is that I believe it works, and that *prevention* is where the real hope is in the struggle against the most feared disease.

So, is there absolute scientific proof that the program in this book will positively prevent disease? No, of course not. Life is seldom that simple. My guess is it would take $50 million, and studying 20,000 patients for twenty years to "prove" such a thing. I recall the forty-year controversy on whether cigarette smoking caused lung cancer! Even today, the struggle continues to keep smoking out of public places, even though, in those forty years of debate, 14 million Americans died from smoking-related diseases. Harvey Diamond's plea is that we not wait for millions of new cases of cancer to occur in the next twenty years, but to do something to prevent them now. Since new scientific evidence and epidemiological studies point strongly to major lifestyle changes that *do* prevent cancer, which the author outlines extensively in this book, one must conclude that Harvey's program will work. At the very least, people who follow it will have more energy, stay slimmer, and feel healthier. At the most, it will prevent a wide variety of degenerative diseases from occurring.

While physicians are still focused on treating cancer already present, Harvey Diamond moves the focus to taking charge of your life so you can prevent it. I am convinced that *Fit for Life: A New Beginning* will become a modern health classic. The book should be read by everyone. It will transform worry and fear into real hope.

—Kenneth M. Kroll, M.D.
Fellow, International College of Surgeons[*]

---

[*]Dr. Kroll received his medical degree from Harvard Medical School and surgical tracking at Stanford Medical Center.

INTRODUCTION

This book is not for everyone. It will be of interest only to those of you who eat.

Ah, yes, food—my favorite subject! What a dominant role food has played, and continues to play, in my life. How about you? It's a good bet that most of you reading this right now are chiming in with agreement, and it's no wonder. Did you know that on average each one of us will consume approximately seventy tons of food in our lifetime? Seventy tons! Yow! No wonder it plays such a dominant role. How could it not? The amount of time, effort, and energy necessary to obtain, prepare, and consume seventy tons of food coupled with the effort of your body to break down that food, extract, and utilize what you need from it, and eliminate the rest, represents a hugely significant portion of your life on this planet. This book will demystify and simplify the entire subject, while empowering you to the point that you know it is you and you alone who is in control of whether you live your life in good health or ill-health.

The common thread woven throughout the book from beginning to end will be the effect of those seventy tons of food on your energy levels, well-being, health, and longevity. Although there has been considerable progress in the collective understanding that food has an impact on the length and quality of your life, it has yet to be fully grasped just how immense that impact truly is.

There are many things that are necessary to live a healthy life, including food, water, air, sleep, exercise, sunshine, loving relationships, cleanliness, and others. Food, water, and air are our most immediate needs, for without any one of them, we soon die. Unfortunately, we don't have direct control over the quality of the air we breathe, but we most certainly have immense control over the food and water we consume.

The purpose of this book is to take you on a journey of discovery. Perhaps for the first time you will discover your wondrous body, how it works, and how the quality of the food and water you consume profoundly affects every aspect of your life as regards your health.

We live in a cause-and-effect universe. Things don't just happen to you. They happen as a consequence of actions you took earlier. Although it may not appear to be so on the surface, absolutely everything regarding your health is happening in an orderly and organized fashion. It can appear that it is haphazard circumstances that bring on ill health, but it is not. Excess weight, lack of energy, pain and discomfort, or serious disease— all are the direct result of either doing something to your body you shouldn't have done, or not doing something that could have prevented a problem before it occurred.

When I first wrote this book in 2000, the overall annual death rate in the United States from the most dreaded of all diseases, cancer, was approximately 552,000. By 2020 that number was approximately 606,520. In 2000, over 40,000 women died of breast cancer a year. Twenty years later, that number has remained about the same.[a] This is in spite of billions of dollars spent on research and innumerable "Pink Ribbon" call-to-action type programs designed to increase awareness and decrease deaths.

What has to be of equal, or greater concern, is the increasingly deteriorating health of our nation's children. We are now seeing what is being referred to as epidemic cases of obesity, autism, ADD and ADHD, asthma, and diabetes in children. Nothing could be a greater or more revealing barometer of the overall state of health and well-being in our country than the ever growing number of sick and sickly children.

Can we do anything about this disturbing situation? Yes, of course we can! But will we? Or will we allow ourselves to continue to be misled and conditioned by those far more interested in making money than in leading you down the pathway to long lasting, good health?

It is crucial we grasp the fact that we are at a crossroads. The decisions we make and the direction we choose to take—right now—will have a massive and lasting effect on the most cherished possession we all treasure most, our health and that of our loved ones. There seems to be a plot afoot, be it intentional or accidental, to keep us ill-fed, poorly nourished, and ever more dependent upon a vast array of pharmaceuticals in order to combat the inevitable result of prolonged inferior nutrition. People are routinely convinced to eat, and to feed their children, foods promoted by slick advertising campaigns that label them as natural and wholesome when they are no more natural and wholesome than a hand grenade.

You might wonder why you should read a book on the subject largely written years earlier. Whether you read a book written last week or last century pointing out that it is the Earth circling the sun and not the other way around, the soundness of the premise remains the same. The principles delineated in this book are as relevant and useful today, if not more so, as the day I wrote them. That is because they deal with biological and physiological aspects of the human body and its relationship to food that is ageless. So whether written last year, last decade, or last century, the principles in the book remain as valid and compelling as any other natural principles that remain true and applicable despite the era in which they are declared. The Earth circles the sun and not the other way around, and the passage of time will never alter that fact. Toss a heavy object from the top of a ten-story building and gravity will pull it downward, and no length of time is going to make that change. The living body is comprised mostly of water; deprive it of water and death will ensue. These examples were as true 100 years ago as they are today. This book is filled with principles associated with the living body that are timeless.

This book is going to take you on a journey of discovery. Perhaps for the first time you are going to discover your wondrous body, how it works, and how the quality of the food and water you consume profoundly affects every aspect of your life as regards your health.

There are two types of treatment people receive: after-the-fact treatment and before-the-fact treatment. After-the-fact treatment is everything done to those who are already suffering from some difficulty or another. The vast, vast majority of treatment in this country is after-the-fact. People become sick and go for treatment to try to recapture their health. After-the-fact is also the entirety of a medical school student's training. Students go to school for many years to learn how to treat sick people after they're sick. We don't go to the doctor when we're well, do we?

Before-the-fact treatment is prevention. There is probably not a subject in existence that is given more lip service and less actual attention than prevention. Only a minuscule amount of research money goes toward prevention while the lion's share—and then some—goes toward after-the-fact treatment. Prevention is not even a subject of study in medical school.

On March 25, 2010, the Associated Press reported that "experts say one-third of breast cancer is avoidable." I'm convinced that the number is significantly higher, and I back this statement up within the pages of this book. Additionally, as reported by Reuters, June 1, 2010, The International Agency for Research on Cancer, relying on data represented to be the most accurate available of the global burden of cancer, states that by the year 2030, cancer deaths worldwide will be nearly double the death rate of 2008. According to the World Health Organization, there were approximately 7.6 million cancer related deaths in 2008. Ten years later, in 2018, there were 9.6 million.[b] Now, mind you, these grim projections are statistics represented by the medical profession and medical thinking. There are those, myself included, who are confident that another, more hopeful outcome, is possible.

It is important for you to know that affirming the idea in the public's mind that the medical profession and medical doctors are the last word and are superior to other healing professions and their practitioners did not come about by accident, nor was it the result of a natural progression based on superior or more effective understanding and treatment.

Most people are not aware of the fact that 100 years ago, the medical profession was not the dominant force it is today. Not by a long shot. In fact, at the end of the 1800s and the beginning of the 1900s the medical profession was merely one among a wide range of healing disciplines all vying for the public's attention. There was, in addition to medicine, chiropractic, Natural Hygiene, naturopathy, hydrotherapy, homeopathy, and a host of lesser-known modalities. What set the medical profession apart from all the rest was its practice of relying upon drugs as its primary tool rather than looking at lifestyle habits, such as diet.

The medical profession at that time was nothing special. It was just one of many professions trying to get a foothold and be noticed. Many people thought medical practice was foolish because all it did was prescribe some drug rather than addressing the cause of the problem. Prior to 1910, medical degrees could simply be purchased through the mail. The medical profession actually had quite a poor reputation.

I personally remember a time when medical doctors actually ridiculed and made fun of people who were so foolish as

Introduction

to suggest that diet had anything to do with cancer. Fortunately, things have changed significantly and the issue is no longer whether or not diet plays a role in a person's state of health; it is now trying to determine the degree to which diet plays a role.

The fact that impeccably reliable and effective methods of prevention and healing are virtually hidden from the general public is a tragedy of immense proportions. It is a form of conspiracy that has kept this lifesaving information from coming to light. Sad to say, there is no bad guy in this piece, no room full of loathsome criminals at whom to point a finger of blame. This conspiracy is so totally pervasive, so completely ingrained in the very "cell structure" of our culture that the conspirators themselves are unwitting. They are not even aware that they are at the center of a colossal injustice that ultimately hastens the demise of not only millions of unsuspecting innocents but also of themselves and their loved ones. This is a conspiracy of ignorance.

The greatest and most effective ally in our quest to achieve the high level of health we all desire is literally right under our noses, yet we ignore it. I am talking about the dynamics of the human body, which is so taken for granted and overlooked as the Godsend it is. What is it that heals a cut finger? Is it the bandage or whatever ointment is applied to the wound? Of course not; it's the body. The human body is self-repairing, self-healing, and self-maintaining.

The focus of *Fit For Life: A New Beginning* is prevention, not treatment. It's what you can do when you're well to ensure that you stay that way. I don't just want to show people what to do after they're sick; I want to show them what to do so they don't become sick. Mark Twain said, "Everyone complains about the weather, but no one does anything about it." That's how I feel about the prevention of disease. Everyone talks about prevention, but frequently that's all it is—talk. The goal of this book is to end all that by giving you something definite, specific, and real that you can immediately start using to ensure that you experience what the Grand Creator had in store for us all along: a healthy, pain-free, and disease-free existence. In other words, vibrant health! Be assured that the exalted state of being to which we all aspire is far easier to attain than you may think.

As my knowledge and understanding has deepened over the years, the need for this book became increasingly obvious to me. I am more convinced today of the worth and value offered herein than I was at its original writing, and all I would ask of you is a fair hearing and a fair trial. See for yourself, as have so many others who have already benefited from its reading, if the information contained in this book isn't just what you have been looking for in terms of a commonsense, logical, and eminently doable approach to achieving long-term, pain-free good health for you and yours.

Our life on this glorious planet is an ongoing journey of discovery, of ourselves and of our surroundings. When you proceed on this magnificent journey in a healthy body that is operating at optimum efficiency, the road before you is made smooth and your life becomes a joyous song of gladness. That is the glory of vibrant health.

Blessings,

Harvey Diamond

Part I

Health Is Your Birthright

ONE

How I Got Here from There

Since the release of *Fit for Life*, I cannot recall the number of people who have asked me how I became interested in the subject, how I learned so much about food and the human body, where I studied, and who were my teachers. And because I am fit and trim, many others have asked me how I can tell people how to lose weight when I, obviously, never had to deal with a weight problem, which is, of course, not the case.

It's been a long and winding road, and if you'll be so kind as to indulge me, I would like to share with you just a bit of the journey. I think you will find it interesting, sometimes painful, sometimes humorous, and frequently similar to some of the experiences you have had.

I was just stepping from my car when the words pierced my ears like an ice pick being driven into them: "Hey, fatty, mind moving your car—that's my space." Ouch! Fatty! Me? The words of this apparent dropout from the International School of Diplomacy served as a most rude awakening for me. How on earth could this guy be calling me fatty when I was using one of my most reliable methods for concealing rolls and folds: a Pendleton overshirt (one size larger than I actually needed) which was *not* tucked in so it would hide my extra girth that I was pretty successfully denying I had anyway. Mr. Sensitive threw a monkey wrench into a very carefully thought-out facade I had constructed, designed specifically to conceal from others what I admitted to myself only in fleeting moments of truthfulness. Doggone it, I *was* fat. I hated being fat. It was the bane of my existence. It was in my thoughts all the time. Should I eat, should I not eat, what should I eat? When? Should I go on another diet? Should I just let it "all hang out" and say, "This is me, take it or leave it?" Why was I so hung up on what others thought of me? Why couldn't I be one of those people who could eat anything that couldn't outrun them and not gain an ounce, instead of the kind that puts on weight just by looking at pictures of food. Why in heaven couldn't I take the weight off on one of these forty-seven different diets I've been on and *keep it off?*

There were two answers to these questions. First of all, I had not yet admitted to myself that I was (and still am) a foodaholic; and second, I was never taught how to eat. I don't mean I wasn't taught how to get food to my mouth. I needed no lessons in that; I was born with a Ph.D. in inhaling food. What I mean is, I was never taught how to eat for my body instead of exclusively for my tastebuds. Were you? Were you ever taught that your body had certain uncompromising requirements *and* limitations? And that if the requirements weren't met, while simultaneously pushing the body beyond its limitations and capabilities, all manner of health problems, not the least of which is excess weight, would dog you all the days of your life? If it *was* taught somewhere along the line, I know *I* was absent that day. The only instruction I ever received was, "Here are the four food groups; eat lots of everything," which I did as though there were a gun to my head. And as a reward, I got to lose control of my body, feel guilty every time I finished another meal or looked into a mirror, go into regular depressions over not being able to get a handle on my "problem," suffer innumerable emotional upsets over having to buy "fat" clothes, feel uncomfortable at the beach, and constantly answer the all too frequent question: "Why don't you lose a few pounds?" Plus, there was the indignity of having to periodically subject myself to one of the many restrictive regimens that was in effect the open admission to the world that I had failed, once again, and had to go on yet one more of these torturous diets, on which I couldn't eat. At least, not what I wanted to eat.

I was so angry all the time, especially at all of those people who seemed able to eat absolutely *anything* that would fit into their mouths and never gain an ounce, while all I had to do was walk by a restaurant, and I put on four pounds.

Does any of this stuff sound familiar to you? I'm sure you have your own tale to tell, but some of this must be striking a chord or you would not be reading another book on diet. So here is my question to you, dear reader: Have you had enough yet? Are you ready now to explore more sensible methods that will bring you long-term results and which have, for far too long, been ignored in favor of the "quick hit" solutions that bring only temporary results at best; or do you need to experience some more pain and discomfort, undertake more drug therapy, or go on just a few more restrictive, regimented diets that suck the joy out of the eating experience before you are absolutely, irrevocably certain, beyond any possible doubt, that *diets don't work?*

If you are ready, *I mean really ready,* to put temporary diets and the like on the junk heap of the past where they belong, and are instead ready to take charge of this area of your life, then read on. You are about to come face to face with what you have been looking for all these long years. In an ideal world I, you, and everyone else would have been taught this information when we were young as a matter of course. We would then have had the *choice* either to make use of it or not. But because of some glitch in the cosmic computer, we were cheated out of what was rightfully ours. So, like unsuspecting innocents, we were thrust into the middle of a dense jungle with no bearings, signposts or guides to direct us, so we had to fend for ourselves as best we could. We have been at a loss ever since, trying this scheme and that, all to no avail. I want you to take solace in the fact that people all over the world, and there are legions of them, have found their way clear of the jungle of hype, false promises, and arduous diets and are living lives dominated by health and well-being. They are pain-free, trim, fit, and happy, without dieting, and you are going to have the opportunity and choice to join their ranks if you wish. It is not a matter of chance whether or not you can be successful; it is a matter of choice, and that choice is yours.

So as you read on, you will find in the pages no magic formulas that restore health while you sleep, no outlandish promises that insult the intelligence, no assurances of ridiculous, unrealistic results that fly in the face of reason, logic, and common sense. No, this is a wake-up call to all those interested in finally doing it right, in accordance with the laws of nature and the actual needs of the body. Not the temporary, "here today, gone tomorrow" measures that have dominated the subject for so long. This way your results can be everlasting, not fleeting.

What you will find is a common sense, logical, and realistic way of life that honors and supports the body and its extraordinary ability to achieve the highest level of health possible when given the opportunity to do so.

HI, MY NAME IS HARVEY AND I'M A FOODAHOLIC

I'm in my mid-fifties and I can't recall a time when I was not a foodaholic. The good news is, I now have control over it, it no longer controls me, for I have learned how to live a life that allows me to fully enjoy all the pleasures of eating the food I like while *increasing* my health and remaining trim and fit.

One of the first questions I invariably ask of audiences I

speak to is, "By a show of hands, how many of you love to eat?" The reaction is *always* immediate and predictable. Along with the usual laughter that ripples through the crowd, the room takes on the appearance of a huge flock of flamingos wildly flapping their wings in unison. The only way I could imagine eliciting a more enthusiastic response would be to ask, "How many of you like to breathe?" (And there are those of you who place breathing on the list of importance right *behind* eating.)

Let's 'fess up: If eating were not a *major* issue in your life, you would likely not be reading this book right now. And hey, how could eating *not* be the significant factor in our lives that it is? It's one of our very first human experiences and we are connected to it at the deepest possible emotional level. Eating isn't only a physical phenomenon, not by a long shot. Our emotional attachment to food has far more of an influence on what we eat and when we eat than most people ever realize.

Before we were born, we were floating in the velvet waters of sublime oblivion in our mother's womb. Absolutely everything was taken care of for us. We were comfortable, safe, secure, and worry-free. All needs were met without our even knowing we had needs. Then, on one fateful day, we were thrust out of our world of cozy, snug security, into the bright, open-air world of reality. What a shocker! All we wanted at that moment was to recapture what had been so familiar, comforting, and friendly for the past nine months. And what is the first thing we experience in this new, unfamiliar, and exposed world of lights and sounds? Mercifully, thanks to the fuller development of gray matter in the collective brains of those whose job it is to assist in this birthing process, we are no longer snatched from the womb and immediately dangled unceremoniously by our ankles and slapped on the rear end. No, we are placed at our mother's breast. *Ahhhh.* In the midst of what is probably the most frightening experience of our lives we are granted a reprieve. There was the familiar heartbeat that had been our constant companion for nine months. We were being held in loving arms, and the crowning glory was a soft, warm breast filled with delicious, nurturing milk. A semblance of normalcy was restored. At that most scary, disturbing and emotionally harrowing time of our tender new lives, all was made well by—that's right—food.

For me, the journey from that day when my fears and discomfort were washed away by my first meal has been dominated by anguishing, craving, loathing, loving, wanting, needing, and obsessing over food. My *entire life* revolves around food. I think about it, talk about it, study it, write about it, and of course, I eat it. *I love food, I love eating.* And it's not only for the physical pleasures, either—the sight of some scrumptious favorite, the many different smells and flavors, the joy of just biting into something I love and having it in my mouth, feeling that sense of satisfaction as the food enters my stomach when I'm really hungry. No, it's so very much more. I can hardly tell you all of the psychological and emotional reasons why one eats food, but it certainly didn't take me long as a kid to realize that there was a whole lot more to food than just staying alive. It was wielded as a reward: "Here's an extra pancake for cleaning up your room." As a punishment: "That's it, you're going to bed without dinner." As a bribe: "Sit quietly like a good boy and I'll get you a big ice cream cone." As a threat: "One more word out of you and no dessert!" It seemed as if every aspect of life could somehow have food associated with it.

I'm one of five children, all boys. Money was not abundant when I was growing up, and the competition with my brothers at dinnertime was fierce. There was usually not enough for everyone to have seconds, so of course, whoever finished his first helpings first got to ask the prized question, "Can I have seconds?" Whoever managed to garner seconds would, of course, wear it like a badge of honor the rest of the night, smirking and strutting around like Napoleon after a successful skirmish. The thing is, we couldn't just blatantly bolt down our first portions as though they might be taken away at any moment in order to be sure and get seconds. That would be too obvious. And my father, who was not a person to mess around with, ran the evening meal like the captain of a well-run ship. He was quite unpredictable with his moods so you never knew when something you did was inappropriate and was going to set him off. If he thought you were slamming down your meal for the express purpose of beating everyone else to seconds, you could be yelled at, cuffed across the side of the head, told you had to do all the dishes alone, or the most dreaded of all, sent from the table without even getting to finish your firsts. No, going for seconds had to be done cleverly, even scientifically. You had to eat as fast as possible without *looking* as if you were eating fast. The speed at which you ate was determined, of course, by how fast the others at the table were eating. So, with eyes constantly darting back and forth to the other plates to see how fast they were being emptied, you measured your intake of food according to the others' progress, timing your last bite to be shoveled in right before anyone else's last bite (remember, they're all doing the same thing), and with mouth full of the last forkful and the tension mounting, you blurt out, "Can I have seconds?"—hopefully without spitting out any of the food in your mouth, which would be a dead giveaway and, despite all your effort, would result in the automatic forfeiture of seconds. I remember my mother's constant refrain to us at the table, "What's the rush, who's chasing you?" That's some picture, isn't it? Need I mention that in our family indigestion was as commonplace after dinner as dirty dishes?

When I now reflect on what I have learned over the years about the importance of one's attitude and environment in eating, I shudder at my experiences during those formative and impressionable years. Food should be blessed to show one's appreciation for it. It should be eaten slowly, so that you can savor the different flavors and not force your body to deal with too much too soon. Ideally, beautiful music and laughter should accompany the meal whenever possible. Happiness, and good feelings should fill the air. In an atmosphere of love, camaraderie, and thoughtfulness, the best that can be hoped for from a meal can be realized. The backdrop of competition, anguish, apprehension, and fear and the absence of joy that permeated my family meals while growing up shaped my attitude toward food in a most unhealthy way that to this day demands my constant attention and awareness to counterbalance. If I don't consciously remind myself to eat slowly, chew my food, and be relaxed, I find myself wolfing down my food exactly the way I did as a youngster. Sometimes I catch myself eating like that when I'm out with friends, and I look up, expecting everyone to be staring at me. Other times, before I catch myself, someone will say something like, "Hungry, Harv?" or, "What did you do, forget to eat today?"

I am still unable to stand in line for food at a buffet or cafeteria. My throat closes up, my heart starts to pound, and I become nervous and irritable. It's as though I'm afraid there won't be enough food left by the time I reach the front of the line, or all the good stuff will be gone. It's horrible. I've tried forcing myself to stand in lines as a means of breaking through this, but so far I've never been able to do it without feeling uncomfortable. It's amazing. It's as though, because of my experiences as a child, these feelings are biologically encoded into my cells. How about you—do you have any habits or patterns around food that seem to take over and you don't know why? Guess what, we all do! This is not to imply that all patterns are negative; some are positive. But we're not interested in the positive ones; they're fine. It's those negative ones we'd like to ferret out, acknowledge, and send packing.

Although there was no food consciousness whatsoever in my house while growing up, and we all ate absolutely whatever we pleased, whenever we pleased, I think it was those dinners described above that were most responsible for spawning my addictive, frenetic, irrational, and obsessive behaviors toward food.

Not *every* dinner was like what I described above. At some there was more than enough for seconds, plus leftovers for lunch or dinner the next day. That's the way my mom would plan it. For example, when she would make fried chicken. Chicken was very inexpensive in the 1950s and was a way of getting a lot of food for relatively little money. So when she made fried chicken for her husband, her five boys, and herself, she made a *lot*. I remember coming into the house, recognizing and following that certain, familiar, mouthwatering smell into the kitchen, and feasting my eyes on what looked like an Egyptian pyramid of fried chicken and my mom toiling away at the stove, adding to the stockpile. It must have taken her hours to complete the task. Those nights dinner was more relaxed and lighthearted because everyone knew they would eat their fill and there would still be some left over. We actually had the time, and took the opportunity, to chew our food before swallowing it. But it was those leftovers that gave rise to another irrational and unhealthy compulsion with food. It was called the "midnight run." I would get up in the middle of the night and raid the icebox. It had to be done with great stealthiness, for getting caught at that particular impropriety guaranteed some major punishment, so it had to be carried out with great patience and care. Each step to the kitchen was measured to create no sound. I had, of course, memorized the places in the floor that creaked when stepped on, and avoided them like shark's teeth. Upon arrival at the refrigerator with anticipation of scoring my prize rising in my throat, I couldn't just yank open the door and dive in. The door had to be opened ever so slowly and steadily so the bottle of salad dressing in the door didn't clank against the jar of pickles, which to me would have sounded like a set of pots and pans thrown down the stairs of the basement. I knew just how to slowly and carefully pry open the door with nary a sound. The big ceramic cookie jar was also a test of one's patience and dexterity. Getting that heavy lid on and off silently was as big a challenge as the refrigerator door. To me it was all like big-game hunting. It wasn't exactly like hunting lions, but it sure as the dickens was as scary.

I recall one night getting the icebox door open, and with my heart pounding like a sledgehammer on an anvil and my mouth filled with saliva, I picked out the fattest, plumpest little thigh in the heap. Just as I was about to sink my teeth into the little beauty, one of my older brothers came up behind me without a sound (he also was well practiced) and whispered, not loud enough to wake anyone but loud enough to practically make my liver shoot out of my throat, "I'm telling." After restarting my heart, I pleaded with him to spare my life and not tell on me. Out of kindness he had me return the thigh to its original resting place and go back to bed with the admonition that he would not tell if I never did that again. At the time I was too young for it to dawn on me that he only happened to be there because he was doing the same thing as I, and probably ate my carefully selected thigh. In fact, it wasn't until years later that I found out that we were all making those midnight runs, including my father. Of course, he didn't have to sneak. He could have kicked the refrigerator over and eaten to the sounds of drums and trumpets and no one would have even *pretended* to hear.

Hoarding was another component of my obsession with food. I would hide candy, cookies, potato chips, packaged pastries, anything that wouldn't spoil, all around my room. They would serve either as sustenance for those times I was banished to my room without dinner or as snacks when my mom wouldn't let me have anything because it would "spoil dinner." Hah! Nothing short of having my teeth knocked out could spoil dinner for me. Besides, to me, meals were merely those times where I continued to eat in what just happened to be a more formal atmosphere.

My favorite snack was potato chips. I could eat an entire bag with ease at any time—before a meal, during a meal, or after a meal. But those darn bags would create a real problem if I was trying to eat them in my room when I was being punished by having dinner withheld. Actually, I became quite adept at reopening the bags so slowly that you couldn't hear a sound. Then there was the decision whether to put the chips in my mouth and let them soften up with saliva so they didn't crunch too loudly, or to go into the closet, bury my face between the clothes, and chomp and crunch to my heart's desire. I had food hidden in so many different places that I would actually forget where some was, then one day I would come across something hidden long before, and it was like finding a buried treasure.

When I grew up, I thought perhaps some of my obsession with food would abate. After all, I had a job, therefore money, and could go where I wanted and do what I pleased. Nope. I thought of food from the moment I awakened in the morning until I hit the pillow at night. Everything I did was done in the context of what, where, and when my next meal would be. In the middle of lunch I was already working out in my mind what I wanted to have for dinner and what snacks I would have before that.

No matter where I went or what I was doing, my main concern was what I was going to get to eat. If I was going to the pier or a theme park, my first thought wasn't, "Oh boy, roller coasters and rides"; it was, "Oh boy, corn dogs and chili fries." If I was going to a movie, I immediately thought not of the movie I wanted to see, but what meal I would sneak in to feast on during the show. To this day I can rarely sit through a movie without at least having popcorn. A movie is not complete without popcorn. If I went to a ball game, the very first thing I thought of was all the hot dogs, peanuts, and ice cream I would down during the three-hour game.

There were no circumstances under which food did not totally dominate my thoughts. If I was in a great mood because of some good thing that happened in my life, all I could think about was having a fabulous meal to celebrate. If I was sad, I ate a big meal of favorites to cheer myself up. If I was feeling guilty or angry, I would eat to feel better.

There was no such thing in my mind as good food or bad food. If I could somehow get it into my mouth, down my throat, and into my stomach, it was good food. As it happened, I rarely, *rarely* ate fruits, vegetables, whole foods, unprocessed foods, or pure foods. It seemed as if the more devitalized, fat-laden, and harmful it was, the more I was attracted to it. And my health reflected that. I suffered from excruciating stom-achaches every day of my life. I was always sucking on a bottle of Pepto-Bismol, which was like drinking liquid chalk and did nothing except make me feel disgusted with myself. Colds and head-aches were as commonplace as hair on a gorilla, and my energy level was pathetic. I didn't exercise, par-ticipate in sports, or do much of anything of a physical nature. The only thing I had enough energy for was getting food to my mouth. There always seemed to be enough energy for that.

At the age of twenty-two, after surviving a one-year stint in Vietnam and coming home and eating with a vengeance I had never known before, my weight topped 200 pounds. That was the crowning insult. I was convinced in my mind that I would never, ever, top 200 pounds, and when I did, I was devastated. Losing weight became an obsession in my life that dominated my thoughts every waking moment. Most of the weight was in my belly, thighs, hips and butt. I hated it. If I went to the beach, I couldn't bear to take off my shirt if there were girls around. I wore baggy clothes thinking it would hide my girth. Shopping for clothes was an ordeal and an embarrassment. Nothing like having only three sizes to chose from: large, jumbo, and "Look out. It's coming toward us." The image I had of myself was of a fat, out-of-control, weak slob. No self-respect, no self-esteem, no self-love.

This is when I entered my dieting years. Oh joy! If there is indeed a hell where people are sent to endure eternal suffering for transgressions too great for forgiveness, it couldn't possi-bly be worse than the three to four years of hell I spent eating weight on and dieting it back off, over and over and over again. Back in those days (late 60s, early 70s) you never heard about the dangers and futility of yo-yo dieting. Today evidence abounds that dieting is a frustrating waste of time because it never addresses the real problem or presents an intelligent, long-term solution to the problem. Diets are short-term, tem-porary solutions that carry within them the seeds of their own failure. And as if that were not enough, yo-yo dieting increases your risk of heart disease. In a study presented at the American Heart Association's Scientific Sessions 2016, researchers discovered that yo-yo dieting could cause women of normal weight to become 3.5 times more likely to die from sudden cardiac arrest.[c]

In the days when I was dieting, you heard *none* of this. Dieting was simply what you did when you got too fat to stand yourself anymore, but the weight *always* returned after the diet was over because you went back to the same old eating patterns that brought on the weight in the first place. That's why *95 percent* of all dieters regain the weight they lost. Each time I embarked on the latest fad diet, I took the frustration of the past failures into it with me. Each one was doomed from the start, yet it was that or nothing. At least I knew if I steeled myself with resolve and went through the ordeal of denying myself food, I would drop 30 pounds or so for a while. But having learned no new tools, I had to watch helplessly as each pound that I'd fought so hard to lose returned slowly but relentlessly. That was the worst part of it, *knowing* that the weight was going to all come back and not being able to do a darned thing about it.

That type of "on again, off again" dieting is a breeding ground for aberrant behavior around food. Invariably, as it got nearer and nearer to the time when I knew I was going to have to start another diet, or start to wear bed sheets with a hole in the middle for my head, I would eat like a man possessed. For a week to ten days I was in "I might as well go for it and enjoy myself—it's going to be a while" mode. It wasn't a pretty sight. I overate anything and everything as though each meal was my last. It was insanity. I actually made myself sick of food (a major feat for me) as a means of hurling myself into the next diet. But that kind of indulgent overeating served only to make it doubly hard on myself. First of all, stuffing myself like that stretched out my stomach so when it emptied I *really* felt hungry, which was hell the first two or three days. Second, I forced myself to go from feasting on anything I pleased to hardly eating at all. The pendulum swing from one extreme to the other was so severe that it was torture. Instead of embarking on a program with an attitude of positiveness and pride that I was doing something healthy and good, I was in turmoil, frustrated and anguished. I thought of one thing and one thing only throughout the length of the diet—*food* and when I would eat again. Nothing else mattered. There were no thoughts that I would be making myself healthier or extending my life or anything like that. No, the only goal I had, the only concern I had, was to lose weight. Every day was long, arduous, seemingly never ending. It was a relentless, nonstop challenge to fill my time and thoughts with *anything* that would divert my attention away from food, if even for fleeting moments. Nothing worked. Imagine stepping on a rusty nail and trying *not* thinking about it while excruciating pain throbs through your foot with every step you take. That's what it was like for me trying not to think about food while I was dieting.

Do you remember when you were young and you thought there might be a monster hiding under your bed or in your closet? You could almost feel its presence? I always dieted for 30 days. I felt if I didn't go 30 days, it wasn't a real diet. Well, for that month I didn't *think* there was a monster around, I knew it, and it wasn't under my bed or in the closet, it was in the bathroom and it was my tormentor yelling at me, jeering at me, laughing at me, ridiculing me, making matters so much more difficult than they already were—the bathroom scale. It just sat there, inanimate, but it ruled my life. I swear, sometimes I thought the damn thing was alive. I would get on it and expect it to yell out something like, "Hey, get off me you big ox." I used to dream about taking a sledgehammer and smashing it into pieces so small and unrecognizable that no one would be able to tell what it was.

My entire day, my state of mind, was totally dictated by the scale. When I could put it off no longer and finally stepped onto it, if I had lost any weight at all, even a single pound, I was filled with enthusiasm and would be positive and upbeat throughout the day (as upbeat as I could be while not being able to eat). If, however, I'd lost nothing or actually put back on a pound or two, I was an ornery, sarcastic, angry wretch with battery acid in my veins, punching walls and kicking furniture all day.

The games I would play with myself and my scale were too much. I didn't want to weigh myself daily because there just wasn't enough progress to show up each day, so I would try to go two or three, or even four days, so I could see some movement. Putting a towel over it or sticking it in the closet was useless, I could "hear" it yelling to me. No, it was all done with mind games. I would promise myself a reward of some kind if I didn't step on it for three days and lost weight when I ultimately did weigh in.

Usually around the third week, when I had dropped weight and my belt size was smaller, I had enough momentum to see it through.

I have the kind of body that puts it on and takes it off very quickly. At the end of my month I would always have lost between 25 and 30 pounds. So I would have some short-lived rejoicing to celebrate my achievement. Why do I say short-lived? Because what is the first thing I would do upon completing a diet in which food has been restricted, measured, and boring? Right—run out of the house like a scalded cat to have some of the very foods I had been denied and dreaming of over the previous month, the very foods and eating habits that created my problem in the first place. By age twenty-five I felt as though I had already finished off my allotted seventy tons and had enthusiastically started in on someone else's.

ENOUGH ALREADY

One day something snapped in me. It dawned on me that the extra pounds I was wrestling with were not the worst of it. I was becoming more and more unhealthy. I was sick with a cold or

some other painful bout of something ever more frequently. So
not only was I fat, but my stomach hurt every day and night.
Truly, no exaggeration, it was terrible. I had migraine headaches
that would leave me curled up in a dark corner swallowing aspirin.
I had so many colds a year, I think I was personally responsible for
Kleenex stock going up. I had blemishes on my face that were
bothersome and embarrassing, and no energy for even the simplest activities so, of course, I never exercised, which com-
pounded my dilemma.

The event that finally motivated me to make some drastic
changes was the death of my father from stomach cancer after
a long and torturous ordeal. I was, of course, convinced that
the same fate awaited me. You see, for years before my father
died of stomach cancer, he regularly complained about violent
stomach pains, the kind I had had my entire life. Up until 25
years old, I felt like I had a red hot poker jammed into my gut.
I lived with regular, unrelenting pain, sucking down bottles of
Pepto-Bismol like water. I never could figure out which was
worse, the pain or that vile liquid chalk concoction that was my
constant companion.

Have you ever seen a movie in which someone bolts up in
bed in the middle of the night with terror in his eyes? Well, that
scene started to play itself out in my life with increasing regularity and it was frightening in a way I cannot fully express in
words. Four, five, sometimes six times a month I would ex-
plode out of my sleep, drenched in sweat, my heart throbbing
in my throat so hard I could barely swallow and the picture in
my mind of what my father looked like near the end of his
ordeal, which, believe me, was as horrific as anything I have
ever seen.

This was truly the nadir of my life. I hurt all the time. I was
overweight. I had no energy. I was more often than not in a
very negative state and far too frequently actually afraid to go
to sleep out of fear of waking up crying or yelling out loud
because of "the nightmare." I think you can see that it was

imperative that I make a change, which is exactly what I did. I knew that nothing short of a drastic, radical change would do, so I cut all ties, got rid of most of my belongings, bought a Volkswagen van named Urge, piled in, and hurled myself out into the world with this prayer on my lips: "Dearest God, please, *please* direct me to what I need to end this suffering. Please, I will do anything." God answered my prayers.

After traveling around searching and basically being open to anything that might bring me some relief, I found myself, through a series of events that could only have been divinely orchestrated, in Santa Barbara, California, talking to someone who would change my life forever. He was introducing me to Natural Hygiene, a phenomenally effective and successful field of study with a 160-year written history that I'd never even *heard* of. He had a library on the subject unlike anything I had ever seen before or since. Much to my good fortune, we became extremely close friends, so much so that we actually shared a house for several years, during which time he counseled and trained me while I devoured his extensive library.

I never was much of a student growing up. To put it bluntly, I hated school. Nothing captured my interest sufficiently to make me *want* to apply myself and study. I was one of those kids who was always being evaluated by my teachers as smart but unwilling even to try. Nothing got through to me. To me, school was that place where I had to go in order to eat my lunch.

My introduction to Natural Hygiene changed all that. I became a motivated and diligent student. This, obviously, was my destiny. I finally found something that genuinely stirred my interest in a deep and profound way. I discovered a thirst I did not even know I had. It was as though I was compelled to study this subject the way a flower is compelled to grow in the sun. It totally consumed me. It was all I could think of. I wanted to learn absolutely everything I could. I knew in the deepest part of me that I had found what I was looking for. I was as excited as when I was a little kid climbing onto my very first shiny new bicycle. Simply put, I took to it the way a dolphin takes to the open sea.

Even my mentor was rather astonished at the depth of my understanding of the subject and how quickly it seemed to become second nature to me. But no one was more astonished than I. My life at this time became a string of excited, fist-pumping *Eurekas!* And as I applied what was the most obvious, common-sense approach to health and well-being that I had ever encountered, miracles started happening in my life. Now I don't know if they were real-life, bona fide, church-ordained miracles, but they were definitely miracles as far as I was concerned.

After all, my life had consisted of pain, and lots of it, on a daily basis. I had created a hell for myself and I was only in my mid-twenties. Then, as if by magic it all ended. As I put into practice what I was learning (and what you will be learning in this book), it was all washed away. My life was given back to me and it happened fast, really fast. It's what I was referring to earlier when I pointed out how magnificently capable the body is in healing itself. Given the opportunity and the proper environment to heal, your body will quickly and efficiently heal itself the same way it heals a cut finger.

The first indication that I had indeed discovered the magic formula and what amazed and thrilled me beyond description, was how quickly and completely *all* pain left me. I could hardly believe it. After so many years of torment, of dealing with and anguishing over pain, it was gone. *Gone.* After suffering from violent, truly excruciating stomachaches for my entire life, they just stopped. (I have not had a stomachache since 1970. I'm beginning to think this really works.) I also had my last migraine. The blemishes on my face completely cleared up. I started sleeping soundly throughout the night, a real blessing. I had such a consistent, high level of energy all the time, some of my friends found me annoying. Plus I dropped 50 pounds. And this all happened the *first month,* so perhaps you can understand why I viewed these healings as miraculous.

I must tell you that during that month of rejuvenation I was dumbfounded at how effectively and efficiently my body fixed itself, given the opportunity to do so. It is what solidified for me, more than any other factor, my belief and enthusiasm for the worth and value of Natural Hygiene. Nothing is more convincing than personal verification. After suffering from so much pain for so many years, decades, it was all so quickly swept away, and for the first time in my life I looked and felt phenomenal. My course for life was set. Words cannot describe the appreciation I felt for this great blessing in my life, and I knew I had an absolute obligation to share it with whoever was willing to listen.

Over the last thirty years there is one question I've been asked more than any other, in fact, probably more than all other questions combined. It was the same question that was on my lips more times than I can recall. Sometimes I would ask it of someone I hoped might know the answer. Sometimes I would just yell it out to the cosmos. I tell you this because as you read through the book and learn what it has to offer, this same question is going to be on *your* lips. The question is, "How on earth is it possible for there to be a system of healing this simple and effective and for it not to be known by the public at large or even the medical community?"

American spend over a trillion dollars a year on health care. That's a one with twelve zeros! That is over two billion, seven hundred million dollars *every single day.* Do you know what kind of an army of sick people must march into doctors' offices and hospitals every day to generate that much money day in and day out? And if you think that money plays no role in why you know all about the medical approach to healing and have never even heard of Natural Hygiene, then you are the perfect candidate to buy some prime swampland in Florida, site unseen.

There was a time in our history when the medical approach to health and well-being was not the predominant health-care system it is today. There was a time when medicine was merely one choice available along with others, such as Natural Hygiene, chiropractic, homeopathy, hydrotherapy, and others. All were vying for the public's health dollar. With the advent of pharmaceuticals, men with immense wealth, power, and influence saw the huge financial potential of drug therapy. Since the medical profession was the only discipline of the day interested in using drugs, these men used all of that wealth, power, and influence to make certain that the medical approach became the official health-care system in the United States. Now mind you, this wasn't done because medicine offered the best hope, the best results, or the most successes in healing. It was done because medicine offered the best potential for generating the greatest financial reward through the marketing of pharmaceuticals. Schools that were willing to teach drug therapy were given funding and thrived. Those not interested in drug therapy did not receive funding and folded. It was as simple as that. Want proof? Is the predominant health-care system in this country one that relies on drugs or not?

Some of you may say, "Oh, Harvey, you're just being cynical or you're suffering from sour grapes or you have an axe to grind." It's not so. What I'm telling you is historical fact, which anyone can go read up on just as I did.

Now I must tell you that there was a time in my life when my attitude toward the medical profession was unrealistic and unfair. You've heard the saying: "Just because there's one bad policeman (or lawyer, or politician, or doctor) doesn't mean they're all bad." And that's true as true can be. One bad apple in the bushel doesn't make them all bad. But for years after my father's horrific death, I considered *all* members of the medical profession my sworn enemies. In fact, six years before the original *Fit for Life* was written, I wrote a book that I self-published and is now out of print called *A Case Against Medicine*. Although it contained a lot of good information that did ultimately end up in *Fit for Life*, it also contained an unrelenting, vitriolic attack against the medical profession. A friend of mine, while living in Los Angeles, once gave a copy of the book to Julie Andrews, the fine actress and wife of producer Blake Edwards. I got the book back with a little note that read, "Who is this angry person?" That was me.

Thank goodness one of the more positive aspects of life here on earth is that, with an open mind and a genuine desire to expand our understanding, we all evolve, grow, and learn. My own journey of learning has brought me to a much more rational and healthy state of mind. My mother once shared a most valuable lesson on life with me. She said, "You don't have to tear down your neighbor's house to build up your own." In other words, I don't have to criticize another person's work in order to make my own work look better. And of course, she was right on target. Her point was that if what I have is of value, it will become apparent to those who make use of it, *irrespective* of what anyone else is doing or saying.

The fact is that no one person and no one group has *all* the answers to what creates optimum health. The subject is simply too vast. If we could somehow measure what we do know about the human body, how it works, and how to best care for it, against what we do not know, it would be like comparing one single star in our galaxy to the billions of stars in the billions of galaxies in our universe. There is no comparison. Those who would declare that only one approach to health care should be followed to the exclusion of all others are saying that for their benefit, not yours.

Understanding this has been instrumental in my own ongoing education. The one thing that we can be absolutely certain of is that what we know is dwarfed by what we don't know. That being the case, can you see that it would be prudent for us all to make use of the best of what each approach to improving health has to offer rather than following only one discipline while entirely rejecting all others?

I can recall numerous occasions when I was doing the talk

show circuit for *Fit for Life* where I was a guest along with one or more other guest authors, each of us there to discuss our books. Invariably we were all told something to the effect of, "Let's point out and discuss your differences." Now I know that makes for a livelier and more interesting show, but how does that format assist the viewers who are tuning in to learn something that can help them live more healthfully? Does it serve the viewers, the very people whom the show is for, to watch a panel of experts fight it out over who's smarter, better, or more innovative? Or does it serve those viewers better to see that panel of experts discussing their areas of common ground? Talking about those aspects of their work where there is unanimous agreement helps viewers, by the end of the show, feel confident that they learned something useful that will improve their lives.

What's my point? Just this—it is arrogance and ignorance of the highest order for one group of practitioners to tear down, ridicule, or declare as worthless an approach to health care based solely on the fact that it differs from their own point of view. Especially when what we know is but a cup of water compared to an ocean of what is yet to be learned. Who can say with unqualified certainty what will or will not work for absolutely everyone.

I want to be as delicate and objective as I can with what I next say because it has to do with the medical profession's role in what I am talking about here. Considering my tendency in the past to blame the medical profession for everything from global warming to tight-fitting shoes, I could see where any attempt I make to give a fair and objective critique could be met with an eye of skepticism. However, I can't allow that to stop me from making some observations that need to be made.

We don't have to embrace every aspect of every discipline, but it only makes good common sense to use the best of each, doesn't it?

So let's take a look at the best of what the medical profession has to offer.

Diagnosis, emergency medicine, trauma care, and surgery—

these are what members of the medical community are educated and trained to do, what they practice and what they're good at. What they are *not* educated and trained to do, what they do not practice and are not good at, is the prevention of long-term, chronic illness. Remember I spoke of before-the-fact treatment and after-the-fact treatment? Before-the-fact means prevention; it's everything you do when well to see to it that you stay that way. After-the-fact treatment is everything that is done after you don't feel well, to remove symptoms, lessen pain, or attempt to cure.

Can you see that the basic function of medicine is after-the-fact-treatment? Rather than focusing on the *cause* of the problem, it focuses on lessening the symptoms of the problem. Just look at the curriculum for a medical student: *everything* is involved one way or another in dealing with sick people, not well people. There are lots of classes on pathology, the study of disease. Do you know there is not even a word in the English language for the study of health? What does that tell you? Besides, when was the last time you felt so vibrantly healthy and so alive and well, so energetic, that you just had to go straight to your doctor's office to be checked out? Never, that's when. That's because medical doctors interact with people *after* their health has been compromised. Is it not the case in your own experience?

Unfortunately, what we have done as a society is look to medical people for answers to questions they are not equipped to provide. Because they are so good at what they *are* good at, we have jumped to the conclusion that they are knowledgeable in *all* areas of health care and that is simply not true. You may know someone who is the most highly accomplished driver in the world. You know if you're in the car with this person at the wheel, you're safe because he or she is the best there is. But a car is only one mode of transportation. As good as this person is at driving, would you trust him or her to pilot an aircraft on which you are a passenger?

Please allow me to present one more choice nugget of information to support what I've been talking about here. I have made and will continue to make throughout this book the point that diet, the seventy tons of food to be consumed in a lifetime, and the quality of water and juices you consume are the predominant determining factors in acquiring and maintaining vibrant health. Hundreds of billions of cells in your body die off every day and must be replaced by new cells. The building blocks for their replacement come from the foods you eat.

The enormous importance of diet in determining our health is no longer a matter of speculation but rather a well established, scientifically substantiated fact of life. There are no longer debates about whether diet plays the immense role we now all know it does, but on what sort of diet is the optimum one for vibrant health.

This being the case, I'm fairly confident you would agree that a person studying to become a doctor could reasonably expect to be taught some nutritional courses at some point in medical school. Yet of the approximately 127 medical schools in the United States, 70 percent do *not* require a single course in nutrition to become a medical doctor. Additionally, at 30 percent of these medical schools, nutrition is not even *offered,* let alone required. It's not available even if you wanted to take it. Nothing more clearly illustrates the fact that the emphasis in medical training and practice is on after-the-fact treatment, not before-the-fact treatment.

If you are looking for after-the-fact treatment, by all means, avail yourself of what the medical approach has to offer. If, on the other hand, you are looking for before-the-fact treatment and wish to learn how to remove the cause of ill health before it can even get started, while laying the foundation for long-term good health, then turn to the approach that specializes in that. It's the approach I've studied for the past thirty years and is the basis of the book now held in your hands.

As I've said, this book is about before-the-fact treatment.

If you're willing to take some simple steps when you are well to ensure that you stay that way, stay tuned: You are about to come face-to-face with how to do exactly that. Always remember that exuberant, vibrant health is your birthright, it is the normal, natural state of your being. Pain, ill health, and disease are abnormal and are not your natural state of being. Contrast this point of view with the following statement made by a person reviewing two medical books back in the 1980s: "From the perspective of the medical profession, healthy people are simply patients pausing briefly on their journey from disease to disease."

The great tragedy of this gentleman's comment is that a staggering number of people have been convinced that his statement is accurate. I cannot tell you how many times over the last three decades I've heard people say things like, "Well, as you get older, you have to expect something to start to go wrong or hurt," or, "It's only a matter of time before something catches up to me." Or, "I've been lucky so far, but sooner or later something's going to get me." Ever hear any of these or ever utter them yourself? These sentiments are classic examples of "stinkin' thinkin'."

For some reason, perhaps from childhood on, people have had the thought implanted in their consciousness that it's inevitable that they will at some point suffer from *something*. Innumerable books have been written on the power of positive thought. Chapter Thirteen of *this* book, "The Mind Matters," delves into that very subject. Among other things, it describes scientifically documented cases of people either making themselves sick or well with their *thoughts*. We're all thinking about something most of the time. Since we're already thinking *something* about our bodies and our health, why not be thinking positive, uplifting, and healthy thoughts rather than negative, depressing, and unhealthy thoughts? It doesn't cost any extra to do so, and the choice is yours. For centuries upon centuries great master teachers have been expressing their view that our thoughts create our reality. I addressed this very thing in a chapter I wrote called, "You Are What You Think You Are," in the original *Fit for Life*, back in 1985.

To understand how you can live your life free of pain and free of disease, you need to cultivate a new way of thinking about your health and your body. Vibrant health is your birthright, it's part of the grand gift of life. The biological makeup of your body is designed to seek out and maintain a consistently high level of health.

It's an intriguing phenomenon about us humans that we all too frequently focus on our differences rather than on our similarities. Who knows how much less strife there would be in the world if it were the other way around. This phenomenon seems to exist in all areas of our lives, be it politics, religion, relationships or diet.

For the overall betterment of humankind in every area of existence, it is time for us to start focusing on what we have in common and not on what we do not have in common. *Fit for Life* offered me the opportunity to learn this lesson well. The original *Fit for Life* is a fantastic book. Both time and its millions of fans have proven this to be so. That's because the information it contains works. But not for everyone. I know of people who have tried the principles in *Fit for Life* based on the enthusiasm of their friends or family members, and even though they followed the recommendations diligently, it wasn't for them.

Check the best-seller lists. It is rare, indeed, for there not to be at least one book on diet and health. Have you ever noticed that no matter how popular or unpopular a certain diet is, no matter how sensible or absurd a program is, there are *always* some people who swear by it? I've seen dietary programs that appeared to be so ridiculous, so nonsensical, so physiologically and biologically unsound, that you'd think no one, truly, *no one* would even go on such a program, let alone benefit from doing so. Yet invariably there will be people who not only follow the diet but thrive on it and say things like, "I've tried every diet to come down the pike and this is the only one that ever worked for me."

The point I'm attempting to make is that we should be ready

to utilize the best of what each approach to health care has to offer.

If at present you are not experiencing exuberant, vibrant health, it is only due to a lack of information as to how to bring it into your life. All knowledge of all things exists right now and always has. The knowledge of how to fly to the moon existed in prehistoric times. It just wasn't found out until the past century. The knowledge of how to experience perfect health all the time exists right now as well, and a lot of people are working to bring that information to light, and no one knows at what point another drop of knowledge from the great unknown will be presented to us.

Some of these drops are on the pages that follow. Clear your mind of preconceived notions and prepare to think a little differently about the subject at hand. Perhaps you'll find what you have been looking for, the same way I did.

TWO

The Clean Machine

If you could be granted one gift, what would it be?

Perhaps your immediate reaction might be to wish for some mind-boggling amount of money, more than could be spent in a lifetime. But upon reflection, most people invariably say that they would wish for uninterrupted, unwavering health. Think about it; to be free not only of any illness whatsoever, but also of the *fear* of developing an illness. After all, what good is a lot of money if you're too sick to enjoy it? If money could buy health, there would be no sick rich people. This book is my attempt to grant you that wish.

Everybody wants to be healthy! And of late, there has been an encouraging surge in the number of people taking personal responsibility for their health, people who have discovered the benefits of upgrading their diets and participating in some regular form of exercise. If you have not yet joined them, this is your time, your opportunity. You can have control over your level of health. You can have a say in the length and quality of your life. You can experience vibrant health. You can! And more and more people are becoming aware of that fact every day. The beauty of this revelation is that taking control and being in charge of your health are not all that complicated. Oh, I know you've been conditioned to believe that they are, but they aren't! And you can turn the tide in your favor almost immediately, depending upon how long it takes you to finish reading this book.

I know that the subject of disease has been complicated to the point of mass confusion and frustration, so I can easily relate to those of you who are skeptical of my claim that you can prevent it just by reading one book. No problem. I can handle skepticism. It's apathy I have to conquer. But if you will give it a chance and just try the suggestions contained here, I will succeed, as will you.

You are going to learn not only *what* you need to do and *why,* but also *how.*

THE KEY TO VIBRANT HEALTH

Understanding the intricacies of the engine of a car and how all the parts interact to make the car run can be a real challenge. On the other hand, anyone who operates or relies on a car quickly learns the fundamentals: Put in fuel and the car will run; to keep the car in good running condition, periodically change the oil. If you don't, the inner workings of the vehicle become silted up with sludge and break down. Neglected long enough, the oil would ultimately become so thick with this sludge that it would become solid. The dirty oil must be replaced with clean oil on a regular basis. There is no amount of *external* cleaning that will substitute for the *inner* cleaning. You can wash, shine, polish, paint, or detail the car until it is the best-*looking* car on the block. But it won't run if the inside of the engine is filthy.

The same holds true for the human body, and understanding this is the key to vibrant health. Like a car, your body depends on fuel (food), which it converts into energy. And as with a car, the inside of your body must also be cleansed regularly or it, too, will become silted up. The result can be all manner of ill health. Just as the oil in your car's engine becomes dirtier and dirtier as time passes, a certain amount of toxic residue is continuously generated in your system as a normal and natural result of the body's biological processes and your daily living habits. This waste must be eliminated from every part of the body.

Fortunately, your body does have the mechanism to expel it. But the body can, under certain commonly experienced circumstances, be overwhelmed. The result is a dangerous and harmful buildup of toxic matter. Where exactly does the waste come from? Some is produced inside the body by the replacement of billions of old cells with new ones every day. The old cells are highly poisonous, and they must not remain in the body. The rest is produced from the food and drink we consume daily. The residue that is not incorporated into new cell structure is waste that must be cleansed from your system.

The cleaner the body is, the better it works. We clean our houses, our tools, our closets, our garages, our stoves, our offices, our clothes, and our cars, and we certainly clean the outside of our bodies. It is peculiar in the extreme that such a simple and essential prerequisite of a healthy life has so consistently been ignored. It's not taught in school. It's not taught in college. *It's not taught!*

Hundreds of billions of dollars are spent annually on health care, but the entire expenditure revolves around expensive screening tests, expensive drugs, and other exorbitant treatments, all of which are designed to address problems after they occur. Sadly, the subject of prevention is given only lip service; and the importance of keeping the body hydrated, cleansed and detoxified is completely ignored.

This is a tragedy of considerable proportion, because detoxifying or "cleansing," the body will do more to lay the groundwork for prevention than practically any other measure you take. If there is, in fact, such a thing as a "secret" or a "key" to health, the cleansing of the inner body is surely it. That is one of the reasons why organizations that attempt to help people overcome drug and alcohol addiction call their programs "detoxification programs." They are literally eliminating their patients' dependence on drugs by cleansing the toxins and drugs from their bodies.

My goal is to help you understand that until the inside of your body is cleansed and rejuvenated, you remain at risk of developing pain and disease. Once this cleansing has been accomplished and you start to enjoy the rewards it brings, you will wonder how you could ever have missed a tool of such inestimable value.

CLEANSE AND REJUVENATE

Isn't it fascinating that whenever the subject of caring for the body comes up, it's always in the context of what should or should not be put *into* the body? Put in more fiber. Don't put in so much fat. Put in pure water. Don't put in chemicals, additives, and pesticides. Put in this or that nutritional supplement. Don't put in salt or refined sugar. Ever notice that there's never a discussion about what should come *out?*

The missing link in experiencing the vibrant health that we all strive for and that still eludes so many is yours for the asking. You merely have to grasp the value of doing what is necessary to clean the *inside* of your body. Whenever you use your car, let the fact that the old, dirty oil must be periodically replaced with clean oil be a reminder that your body deserves at least as much attention. Let the letters C-A-R come to stand for something new: Cleanse And Rejuvenate. And don't worry, by the end of the book you'll have all the tools you need to minimize the harmful buildup of waste in your body. You will see exactly how to accomplish the regular Cleansing and Rejuvenation I so emphatically suggest.

ENERGY—THE ESSENCE OF LIFE

In order to accomplish the goal of cleansing, or in order to accomplish any goal, for that matter, there is one decisive element that must always be present. It is the one commodity that everyone knowingly or unknowingly wants, the one that will allow you to do everything you wish to do in life, the one that you can never have too much of. No, it's not money. It's energy! Energy is the very essence of life. When it is plentiful, all things are possible. You feel you are omnipotent. When it dwindles, life becomes an ordeal, and you find yourself at the mercy of all the forces around you. When energy is completely absent, life is over.

Amazing stuff, this energy. You can't see it or hold it in your hands, but you sure as heaven know when someone around you has it. And you certainly know when *you* have it. As human beings, we literally are energy systems. The truth is, there is not one activity or process of the body that can or will be performed without energy. Everything that you do and everything that your body does requires energy.

Back to the car analogy. What good would your car be to you if it had no engine? What good would the engine be to you if you had no car to put it in? Cleansing and energy levels are that interrelated. So much so that we are practically dealing with a catch-22 in that we must have energy to cleanse and we must cleanse to have more energy. Just as in its unfathomable wisdom the body allots energy to the circulation of your blood and the constant beating of your heart, it is also acutely in tune with the need to regularly cleanse itself of deleterious waste and it automatically allots or conserves a certain amount of energy to do this.

"CARE"

Throughout nature, all forms of life herald the spring season with signs of rebirth. Flowers bloom, hibernating animals awaken, new life appears everywhere. And spring also invokes the age-old tradition of "spring cleaning," when we go from the attic to the cellar getting rid of the old and starting fresh. This commendable industriousness must also be extended to the most precious possession of all: your body. I am sure that at some time you have thought of a real spring cleaning for your home. Care about your body in the same way. When you care for your body, it cares for you. Your caring is best exemplified by allowing your body to function at its greatest level of efficiency. And that is only possible when it is cleansed of anything that might interfere with its smooth operation.

Isn't the word "care" a beautiful word? It can be used to express so much feeling or concern:

"I care about what you are feeling."
"My mother shows such care to everyone."
"She took such good care of me."
"I care for you."
"I promise to take care of everything."

There is something about the word "CARE" that brings to mind positive feelings: help, empathy, compassion, concern, love.

I now wish to introduce you to a brand-new meaning for the word "CARE," the meaning that is a major reason that this book was written. I have expressed how crucial it is in your quest for vibrant health to cleanse and rejuvenate the inside of your body. I have also touched on the pivotal role energy plays in the cleansing process. Remember the observation that C-A-R are the three first letters of Cleanse And Rejuvenate? Now take the "E" from the beginning of the word "energy" and put it at the end of the word "CAR." You have CARE: CLEANSE AND REJUVENATE ENERGETICALLY. That is the new meaning of the word "care" that will ensure for you a long and healthy life. CAREing for your body is the best possible health insurance you'll ever have. This process that I call CARE is the ultimate tool in preventing disease and eliminating pain, while invigorating your entire life.

Understanding the dynamics of how toxins are stored up and removed from your body is the key to understanding the importance of making CARE an integral part of your lifestyle.

WASTE MANAGEMENT

The accumulation and elimination of a considerable amount of toxic waste matter in the body are physiological facts of life. The question is: Where does all this waste come from? And where does it go?

The body is essentially a machine that requires fuel, turns that fuel into energy in order to carry out its many functions, and generates waste in the process. Just like a car. There are two kinds of waste produced in the body. The first is generated entirely from internal sources; the second from external sources.

When I speak of internal waste, I am referring to the consequences of cell regeneration. Literally hundreds of billions of old cells are replaced with new cells every single day! The worn-out, spent cells are toxic and must be eliminated, and the body uses the eliminative organs—the bowels, bladder, lungs, and skin—to get rid of them. This cell replacement process is an automatic phenomenon. It is as spontaneous a process as the circulation of blood or the digestion of food. We have no control over this internal waste production.

What we do have some control over is the waste generated as a result of what we put into our bodies. This waste is the end product of all the metabolic activities occurring in every cell of the body. Every cell is a miniature "body" in its own right, taking in what it requires and excreting its wastes. Problems arise only when the buildup of toxins exceeds what the body can eliminate via the eliminative organs. It's very simple. If, on a daily basis, more toxins are produced than are removed, the excess remains in the body, where all manner of problems can develop because of it.

How sad that the prevailing opinion of traditional medicine ignores the need for inner cleansing. This tragic oversight results in all the clogged, choked-off, and self-poisoned bodies that are unnecessarily treated with drugs and surgery. If only it were true that our bodies do not get dirty, and that cleansing is not an issue! But it is an issue and the proof is all around us.

For example, millions of people are walking around with distended abdomens due to a buildup of waste that has not been eliminated. They spend a fortune on laxatives each year because they cannot have something so natural and basic as regular bowel movements without drugs. Millions of others suffer from skin problems or high blood pressure. Others have sinus and respiratory problems. All these conditions are the result of dirty bodies.

It would be nice to think that all wastes are removed from the body, but the body can get rid of only so much. Think of a bathtub full of water. If you pull the plug but leave the water running and more is going into the tub than is leaving it, what is the only inevitable result? The tub will overflow. When this happens inside the body with toxins, it spells pain and disease. If it were true that the body always rids itself of harmful or inappropriate substances, it is unlikely that nearly a million people a year would be losing their lives due to clogged arteries. These arteries are not clogged with good intentions! They're clogged with sticky, toxic waste matter that the body *wanted* to get rid of and *should* have gotten rid of but couldn't.

If you lived in a house in which you did not clean the floors, did not empty the garbage, did not wash the bedding, did not wash the dishes or the windows or periodically dust, you could survive there, but what would it be like? Perhaps you are saying right now, "Who in their right mind would ever let a house go like that?" But far too many people are unknowingly allowing this kind of neglect right inside their own bodies.

The principles of CARE presented in Part II are going to make sure that you are not one of those people. The program is designed to allow your cleansing mechanism to operate at optimum efficiency so you will not suffer from pain and disease, consequences of a body overwhelmed by toxins.

THREE

What's in a Word?

I make my living with words, writing them and speaking them. I love the fact that the right words in the right combination can trigger all manner of emotions. Some words can make you feel warm and fuzzy, like the word "love." Other words can make you feel apprehensive, like the word "crash." You think of something sweet and pleasant with the word "rose." But the opposite is brought forth with the word "skunk." Some words have different meanings depending on how they are used even though they are spelled and pronounced the same way. Take the word "terrific." You can use it to describe something horrible and terrible, or something wonderful and grand. There are words that can mean different things to different people, depending on their personal experiences. But there is one word that has basically the same effect on everyone and there's nothing good or positive associated with it. It's a word that most people don't want to hear, utter, or think about, and here I am faced with the need to bring it up to you in order to fully explain the premise of this book. I don't mind telling you it's a big challenge for me to do it in just the right way.

I know I've already told you several times that for you to receive the most and best of what this book has to offer, a new way of thinking was the key. I can tell you here and now, that your ability to think differently will be stretched to the limit as it relates to this word I'm referring to. "All right already," you're thinking, "what's the word?" Cancer. There. I spit that bad boy out. What came up for you when you read that word? Anything good?

What if you were to learn that cancer is not even what you thought it was? What if all your life you were led to believe it's something other than what it actually is? You know, there are numerous instances throughout history where the entire world thought something only to find out the exact opposite was true. The entire population had to alter its thinking. Textbooks had to be rewritten. I'll give you the most classic one I can think of. There was a time when *everyone* was convinced that the Earth was the center of the universe and the sun revolved around it. And when certain scientists and astronomers began to declare that the exact opposite was true, they were harassed, villified, and generally made to feel uncomfortable—in jail! At that time it was considered to be blasphemy and the blasphemers were, to put it mildly, not well tolerated.

I am definitely not going to attempt to convince you that cancer is a good thing. But I can tell you that most people don't understand even the most rudimentary aspect of its nature. Most people look at cancer as some monster that crawls up out of hell and eats away at its victims until there's nothing left except the funeral. We fear what we don't understand and people's immense fear of cancer is right on par with their level of misunderstanding of what cancer actually is.

TO UNDERSTAND HEALTH,
UNDERSTAND CANCER

Have you ever heard the statement, "Every stick has two ends"? It means the same thing as, "There are two sides to every coin." In order to understand one side of an issue, the other side also has to be examined. And that is most certainly the case here. I recall hearing the following statement many times. "Knowing what you *don't* want is every bit as important as knowing what you *do* want." How about you? For example, someone trying to figure out what profession to go into might be told by a trusted adviser, "Figuring out what you don't want to do for a living will help you figure out what you do want to do."

In order to ascertain what vibrant health is and how to attain it, we must examine what is at the very opposite end of the spectrum. In this case, "the other end of the stick" is *the* most classic lifestyle disease there is: cancer. The vast majority of people, I have found, don't have the vaguest idea what factors lead to cancer. When you *do* know what those factors are, it is then an easy matter to avoid them.

When you learn exactly what cancer is and exactly how it occurs (which you will very shortly), it becomes obvious how to prevent it. By learning how to adopt a lifestyle that results in vibrant health, which is exactly what you will learn from this book, you automatically make cancer an impossibility. Obvi-ously, the two cannot coexist.

Cancer is America's Number 2 killer (heart disease is Number 1), and takes more than half a million lives every year. The world over, cancer is a major health problem, one that has become progressively worse every year for about the last century. A predominant reason for this is that the nature of cancer is invariably misinterpreted and misunderstood. You see, *cancer is not the problem, it is the end result of the problem.* And because this simple truth has been so universally misunderstood, billions upon billions of dollars have been squandered in a futile attempt to treat and/or cure people *after* it's too late and they are in jeopardy of losing their lives. Worse yet is that so many millions of people suffer immeasurably before ultimately dying *unnecessarily* from something that could have been prevented in the first place. In fact—and this may turn out to be one of the most controversial statements I have ever put in print—I am hard-pressed to think of any malady of the human body easier to prevent than cancer.

Late in 1998 there was a huge rally in Washington, D.C., called "The March: Coming Together to Conquer Cancer," which drew 150,000 people. They made the point that 1,500 people died on the *Titanic,* seen to be such a huge tragedy, and that number of people die *every single day* from cancer. The 150,000 people were demanding that, "The nation make *curing* the disease its top health-care priority!!¹ No no no *no NO!* We must make *prevention* the top priority.

If someone is in a devastating auto accident, it's done. That's it. There's no curing it, the damage is already done. Had that person been better instructed on how to drive defensively, be ever alert to expect the unexpected and take no unnecessary risks, there's a good chance that the accident could have been avoided before it happened. I'm going to show you how to prevent becoming sick before it happens. You see, being sick, or experiencing pain, represents the preamble to cancer. The information contained in this book will help you fully appreciate and understand that pain, discomfort, and ill health are the first, faint warning signs that something is not right and must be changed or the situation will worsen. At that point in time the appropriate measures must be taken to remove the cause of the pain and discomfort. If, instead, you ignore the cause or take drugs to silence these warnings, then you are taking those first fateful steps onto a path that, with continued neglect, can lead to that most dreaded of diseases—cancer.

By the time you finish this book you will not only know

how to prevent cancer, but also how to prevent any sort of pain or illness. A Louis Harris poll revealed that people's Number 1 health complaint is pain. You will learn exactly what pain is, the extremely important role it plays, how to remove it, and how to prevent it from ever recurring. The means by which this is accomplished is so obvious and so simple it absolutely astonishes me that it has been missed for so long.

The way this is achieved is not by studying cancer—the effect—but by studying the factors that bring on cancer—the cause.

Remember that the universe operates under the law of cause and effect. Things don't just happen, they happen for a definite reason. There is an action and then a reaction. In this instance, the things we do, knowingly or unknowingly, to jeopardize our health are the actions, and cancer is the reaction. Studying cancer, which is the end result of prolonged abuse and neglect, would be like rushing out to lock your garage door after someone has already driven off in your car.

In order to obtain the maximum benefit from this book, it is crucial that you understand that when you focus on the reaction instead of the action that caused it—when you focus on the effect instead of the cause that brought it about—then you are forced into that unenviable position of having to focus on after-the-fact treatment instead of prevention, because it means you're already sick and it's too late for prevention.

It's what I have been referring to when I said I wanted to give you a brand-new way of thinking about health and disease. The old way of thinking is to wait until you're sick and then battle your illness with the latest weapon—in other words, treat disease. The new way of thinking is to learn what factors cause you to become sick, and then avoid them—in other words, prevent disease. And you are going to learn how to achieve that goal by studying and learning about causes, not effects. It is likely that some of your beliefs will be challenged by what you read here. All I am asking for is a fair hearing. Read what I have to say and I promise, you will not be disappointed.

THE WAR ON CANCER

Even though cardiovascular disease regularly kills more people a year than cancer, ask anyone which is more feared, and you will inevitably hear cancer. But very few people know what cancer is. Do you? Ask your friends if they know what cancer is and they'll all say something like, "Of course I know what it is, who doesn't?" But when it comes right down to it, people don't know. They know the *results* of cancer and its treatment, but unless they work in the health field in some capacity, they do not know what it actually is. And guess what? *Those* people, the researchers, the scientists, the ones who are supposed to know, don't know either. That's right. Oh, there are suppositions, presumptions, inferences, theories, and hypotheses galore, but when you get right down to it, the "experts" are still trying to fully understand cancer.

In 1971, then-President Richard Nixon inaugurated the "War on Cancer" with the National Cancer Act. The National Cancer Institute's budget was more than doubled for 1972,[2] and it was confidently proclaimed that we would have a cure by America's two-hundredth birthday celebration in 1976.

The first major assessment of the "war" came fourteen years later. In 1971, one in four Americans developed cancer. Fourteen years later, this statistic increased to one in three.[3] In 1971, two in three families were affected. Fourteen years later, it was three in four. In 1971, the mortality rate, which is truly the most important number of all, was one in six. Fourteen years later, it had become one in five—a 22 percent increase.[4]

Dr. John Bailor, a biostatistician at Harvard, was editor of the *Journal of the National Cancer Institute* and had worked at the Institute for twenty-five years. In 1986, in the *New England Journal of Medicine,* he co-authored a study of the results of the fight against cancer from 1950 to 1985.[5] He wrote that the data provided no evidence that some thirty-five years of intense and growing efforts to improve the treatment of cancer had much overall effect on the most fundamental measure of clinical outcome—death. Indeed, with respect to cancer as a whole, we have slowly lost ground. Incidence of cancer is also increasing, suggesting a failure to prevent or control new or current causes of cancer.

The researchers concluded, ". . . some thirty-five years of intense efforts focused largely on improving treatment must be judged a qualified failure." It doesn't get any clearer than that. In 1997, another article by Dr. Bailor in the *New England Journal of Medicine* called again for more focus on prevention. In this article, he gave yet another dismal report on the cancer situation in the United States.

Today, almost thirty years since declaring "war" on cancer, with over $35 billion spent on research (that's only federal money; much more than that was spent in private money), $1 trillion spent on treatment, and over 8 million deaths, we are no closer to a "cure" now than we were then. It is blatantly obvious that the best and smartest minds medical science has to offer have been confounded and bewildered by cancer. When CNN correspondent Carl Rochelle asked if we are losing the battle against cancer, Dr. Samuel Epstein of the University of Chicago Medical Center answered with sobering directness, "Oh, I think we've really lost the fight against cancer. There have been major increases in cancer rates over the last four decades."[6]

Since Richard Nixon declared the war on cancer in 1971, billions have been spent on cancer research in the United States, yet the overall mortality rate is 8 percent higher. This has led cancer experts to tell Congress that the war against cancer has stalled, and that without major changes, it will become the nation's *top* killer in five years.[7]

Good grief! With all the headlines regularly splashed before our eyes proclaiming all the advancements being made in "the battle"; with all the technological progress that has supposedly been realized; with all the billions and billions of dollars being spent; the latest news, as we cross from one century to the next, is that things are worse than they've ever been and are expected to get even worse.

Consider the following, taken from the *London Daily News:* "A man of middle age would have difficulty in numbering the cures for cancer which have appeared and disappeared in his lifetime. Millions of animals have been tortured throughout the world to find the cure of a malady which has been steadily increasing for 50 years. Flare headlines in the daily newspapers once more announce, or at least suggest, that we are on the eve of the most sensational medical discovery of the age." Sound familiar? If you read that in your morning newspaper today, would you give it more than a passing glance? Well, these words were written February 1, *1924!* Over three-quarters of a century later, we're still hearing the same old stuff.

WHAT CANCER REALLY IS

The seriousness of these grim facts makes it all the more essential that we focus on prevention. And since prevention is precisely what this book is about, there is no need for me to go into an overly technical explanation of what cancer is. I will briefly describe the nature of cancer, but only to the extent that it will help you understand how and why the principles outlined in this book will help you achieve vibrant health. I promise you, it will be the simplest, most easy-to-understand description you have ever read.

Many people might think that demystifying and simplifying cancer is a daunting task. The subject has been buried beneath such an avalanche of jargon that most people perceive it as too complicated, bewildering, and obscure, and they give up on trying to understand it. They decide that the subject is best left to the professionals who can wade through the quagmire and make some sense of it all. Wrong. That kind of thinking may be convenient for the professionals, but it keeps you out of the decision-making process that could affect your very life.

When it comes to health care, your body, and medicine, there are two ways you can be given information. One is in an incomprehensible, convoluted way; the other is with straight-forward, unencumbered talk. For example, I could tell you that I have antecubital and retropopliteal urticaria with pruritus, or I could simply say my arms and legs itch. I could tell you I'm experiencing orthostatic hypotension, or I could tell you I'm dizzy. See the difference? Guess which approach the professionals have used to tell you about cancer? No wonder you think it's a perplexing subject that you could never understand.

There are people out there who will not accept my contention that cancer, a subject which has been misunderstood and overly complicated, is actually quite a bit more uncomplicated and understandable than we've been led to believe. It all depends on which point of view you choose. The medical explanation, which is likely the only one you have ever been exposed to, is quite different from that of Natural Hygiene, the field of health care I chose to study.

Let's begin where we agree. Your body is made of cells. Lots of them. One hundred trillion of them. (That's a one with fourteen zeros!) Absolutely every part of you is made up of cells, joined together to form skin, bones, muscles, organs, teeth, hair, fingernails, vocal cords, eyeballs—*everything*. All these cells, right down to the very last one, are under the juris-diction and direction of the brain. The cells in your body are not running around unilaterally, going where they want to go and doing what they want to do. It's not as if a liver cell could say, "I think I'll be an eyeball cell today and see what's going on. It's too dark down here." No. Each and every cell, down to the last one, does what it is instructed to do. In my opinion, the most astounding fact in all of the universe is that every last one of these hundred trillion cells is constantly sending messages to the brain asking for instructions, as it were, and remarkably, the brain receives and answers each and every message. The trillions of messages are sent up and back twenty-four hours a day, ceaselessly, and the myriad functions of the body are performed with pinpoint perfection, all *simultaneously!*

Each cell is like a soldier in the army awaiting orders. Every activity, no matter how minuscule, is performed under the direction and supervision of the brain. The process is orderly and predictable. No cell ever does *anything* unilaterally.

Well, as is the case with most things in life, there are exceptions. The exception here is . . . cancer. A cancer cell is a normal cell so deranged by toxic substances that it loses contact with and is no longer controlled by the brain. It has literally been driven "crazy" by poisoning, and it is "out there on its own." Whereas normal cells divide and stop dividing after a certain fixed time, cancer cells do not. Instead, they proliferate in a disorderly fashion. Two normal cells placed on a slide will stop growing as soon as they touch each other. Cancer cells, in the same conditions, keep on growing; wildly, and out of control. In most cases of cancer, unrestrained cell growth leads to the buildup of tumors which will consume and destroy normal cells.

Obviously, what all the world wants to know is what drives the normal cells crazy. Figure that out and you've figured out cancer. According to the concepts of Natural Hygiene, it is the toxins that normal cells are relentlessly forced to come into contact with for years on end that finally drives some of them crazy. And you learned exactly where these poisonous toxins come from in the previous chapter. Cancer is the end result in a long, pathological evolution that had its beginning long before any chemical signs of cancer showed up. In other words, what is crucially important for you to realize is that *cancer does not attack, it evolves.*

There is a widespread misconception about cancer which I must clear up right now: Cancer is cancer—regardless of what part of the body it affects. A cancer cell is a cell gone crazy and that can happen anywhere in the body. The only thing that differentiates one type of cancer from another is its location, not its nature. The area of the body in which cancer develops is incidental to the fact that it did actually develop. People talk of breast cancer or colon cancer or prostate cancer or cancers in other areas of the body as though they were all separate and distinct diseases. They aren't. Again: Cancer is cancer regardless of where it appears in the body. If people live their lives in such a way that the cells in their bodies are forced to contend with a relentless barrage of toxins for years on end, then there is a strong likelihood that some cells somewhere in the body will go crazy.

Where that happens isn't the most important thing. *Why* it happens is the issue.

To say that breast cancer is a different disease from prostate cancer, which is a different disease from colon cancer, would be exactly like saying that rain, snow, ice, sleet, frost, dew, and hail all have separate and different essences when, in fact, they are all water in different degrees of consistency. Rain and snow may be different in appearance but they are just water in different forms. Breast cancer and prostate cancer may be different in appearance, but they are just cancers in different forms.

In my local newspaper there was an article describing the experiences of three people who had cancer. One woman spoke of her "three kinds of cancer."[8] She lost a lung to cancer in 1983; she lost a breast to cancer in 1986; and she had a skin cancer excised in 1992. The article stated that she took responsibility for getting the lung cancer because she had smoked for thirty-four years. However, in her words, "But my breast cancer—what did I do to get breast cancer? What did I do?"

What she didn't realize is that smoking, which in my opinion is the single most toxic offense against health in existence, affected her whole body, not only her lungs. Of course, the lungs would probably be the first area of the body to be affected by smoking, but it is a person's entire lifestyle that determines whether or not cells are driven crazy. Something as inherently poisonous as smoking affects *all* the cells of the body, not only the cells of the lungs. The woman's smoking was a factor, a major factor, in her cancer of the lungs, cancer of the skin, and cancer of the breast. Because of smoking, together with other negative lifestyle habits, her body simply started to break down at its weakest points.

Cancer will never just happen. It will inevitably be the result of causes that were not removed over a very long period of time. Cells are driven crazy at a very slow pace. You don't go to bed one night and wake up in the morning with cancer. It takes one year for a single cancer cell to become twelve cells. At that rate of growth, it will take six years for the cancer to be the size of a pencil point,[9] and about ten years to even be detectable.[10] At that point, it is one centimeter, about the size of a pea. This is why I say that cancer is the classic lifestyle disease. In the next chapter you will see exactly how this is so. Traditional therapies of surgery, radiation, and chemotherapy attack the problem at the end stages of its growth, after the fact. It is attacking the effect while ignoring the cause. If a person has a tumor or an organ removed and goes right back to the same lifestyle that brought on the problem in the first place without addressing the cause, health will not be restored and this individual's cancerous condition will then "come back." You will hear, "You've relapsed," or "It's returned," or "We must not have gotten it all." It didn't "come back," it never left! Removing a prostate gland or cutting off a breast without removing the *cause* of cancer and thinking that the cancer will not return is like thinking that by picking all the apples off a tree, no more apples will grow.

When the toxic conditions that resulted in abnormal cell growth are removed, then and only then will health begin to be restored. This is provided, of course, that the condition has not advanced so far that irreparable harm has been done. Irreparable harm means that negative conditions existed without letup for so long that the diseased state finally resulted in cells being driven crazy. If that cancer metastasizes, which means it breaks loose from the original site and spreads to other areas of the body, then, obviously, preventive measures are futile and another course of action must be undertaken. This, of course, is the downside in all of this. There is an upside as well.

Remember the upside: Cancer takes some ten years to develop. Disease has seven distinct stages, and if the cause of the problem is corrected during any of the first six stages, health will be restored and cancer, the seventh stage, will not develop. In other words, you have years to turn things around and do what is necessary to prevent cells from ever being driven crazy. Plus, your body is always ready to do its part.

THE SELF-HEALING BODY

Natural Hygiene teaches us that the body is always, *always* striving for the very highest level of health possible. The human body is self-repairing, self-healing, and self-maintaining, and as a matter of course, persistently marshals its forces in a tireless quest to achieve and maintain health. Health is the normal, natural state of your body. Ill health is abnormal and unnatural. When you are healthy, your body automatically directs its efforts toward maintaining that state. When you're in a state of ill health, the body diligently strives to restore health. Every one of the trillions of functions your body performs every day and night without letup are performed as part of its never-ending effort to procure and preserve health.

The same way a ball full of air will shoot up to the surface if submerged in water and then let go, your body strives for optimum health under any and all circumstances. Once the ball is released when underwater, it can do one thing and one thing only—get up to the surface in as direct a route and as quickly as possible. It doesn't hesitate, move side to side, stay down, or stay put; it makes a beeline for the surface. It can do nothing else. Your body, in its quest for health, is the same. It is always striving to achieve health in the quickest, most efficient way.

The ball can only be kept underwater if it is held down. Your body can be prevented from achieving its goal of vibrant health only if it is forced to handle more than it can contend with and its defenses are overwhelmed. Even then, it does not give up trying. As long as the body is alive, it is striving for health.

Fortunately for us all, the body has a built-in mechanism that warns us when its health is in jeopardy. The more critical the problem, the more intense the warnings. Unfortunately, most people do not realize that their bodies are trying to get their attention to alert them of impending danger. Because the warnings are not recognized as such, they are either ignored or masked with drugs. What starts out as a situation that could have been corrected before becoming life-threatening is allowed to progress and deteriorate, all too frequently culminating in cells being driven crazy.

During the first six stages of disease, the body initiates these warnings, and it is crucial that you don't miss them by failing to realize what they are and what they mean. If you are able to recognize the warnings for what they are, you can take the appropriate measures to protect yourself and prevent the end result of continued neglect—disease.

The next chapter describes the seven stages of disease and the warning signs they produce. Read it carefully. More than once if need be. Familiarizing yourself with the information it contains has the potential, not only to save you untold heartache, anguish, pain, and suffering, but also to save your life. It is one of the prime factors in understanding how to achieve vibrant health.

FOUR

The Seven Stages of Disease

Vibrant Health	1	2	3	4	5	6	Cancer

You are looking at the "two-ended stick" described to you earlier. We all wish to be on the vibrant health end of it, obviously. It is the goal and purpose of this book to help you learn how to achieve this.

Have you ever heard yourself say of someone's illness or death, "I can't believe it, he was so healthy" or "I just saw her the other day, and she looked fine."

Be very clear about something: Disease never, ever just sneaks up on people and strikes them down. It doesn't happen that way. It takes a long time and a great deal of neglect and abuse of the body for disease to finally occur. From the first stage of disease to the seventh (i.e., cancer), many years may elapse. At any stage, you can stop the disease's progress, and simultaneously end all the aches, pains, and ill health which were the body's warning signs that changes needed to be made or the situation would deteriorate further. By familiarizing yourself with the seven stages of disease and their warning signals, you put yourself in control of your health. *You* are in charge, not outside influences.

As you familiarize yourself with the seven stages, I want to impress upon you the fact that these stages don't come into being quickly. It doesn't happen in seven days or seven weeks or seven months. Each stage progresses slowly. You can be dealing with each stage for years, sometimes many years, before one stage will progress to the next.

During any of the first six stages, if the *cause* of the problem is removed, pain stops, the disease process stops, and health returns. If drugs are employed to quell the discomfort (the usual course of action), the cause remains unchecked, the disease process continues (even though the drugs may mask the pain, giving the false impression that the situation is improving), and the next stage of disease inexorably occurs.

ONE: ENERVATION

The first stage of disease is enervation. The word "enervation" comes from the word "energy." Energy is the essence of all life. Your very existence depends upon how much energy is available at any given time to carry out all of the functions of your body. Enervation is a condition in which the body is either not generating sufficient energy for the tasks it must perform, or the tasks the body must perform are greater than the normal energy supply can cope with. When this occurs, the body becomes impaired and generates even less energy. In fact, all of the body's functions become impaired, and this includes the processes of elimination of the toxic by-products of both metabolism and the residue of the 70 tons taken into the body. A certain amount of toxins in the body is totally natural. Problems arise when there are more being produced than are being eliminated. Not only does this situation result in the further inability of the body to restore depleted energy, but it also allows the body to become overladen with toxic material. Since energy is restored when you sleep, the first warning sign that you are becoming enervated is that you will become tired and sluggish or require naps during the day and/or more sleep at night.

Of all the symptoms that signify the body is in some kind of distress and is trying to correct it, there is one that will be seen more often than any other: loss of appetite. Nothing is a more reliable indicator. Digestion requires a significant output of energy. When energy is needed to perform some immediate healing function, the wisdom and intelligence of the body instinctively knows to decrease your desire for food. This frees the energy that would have been used for digestion and diverts it to the greatest area of need. That is why practically every list of symptoms for mankind's ailments includes loss of appetite. It can be seen here in Stage 1, and in all the subsequent stages as well. Enervation leads directly to the second stage of disease.

TWO: TOXEMIA

Toxemia (also referred to as toxicosis or autointoxication) occurs when the uneliminated toxic material described above starts to saturate the blood, lymph nodes, and tissues of the body. The body recognizes that this situation must be remedied and, in an attempt to cleanse itself and maintain its health, initiates a flushing out of the toxins. Expect two results when this happens: first, more recognizable warnings in the form of discomfort; and second, an ever greater drain on the body's energy supply. If you are also overworked, under stress, or getting insufficient rest and sleep—all energy sappers—the feelings of tiredness and sluggishness become more pronounced. When the level of toxemia has reached the point where the toxins must be eliminated, the next stage of disease develops.

There is one classic, universal symptom that is the most obvious indication that toxins have reached the point where the body must remove some before they start to do damage. It can be seen in this second stage of disease and in all of the subsequent ones. As I said, it is the most obvious example that the body is in the mode of trying to cleanse itself of toxins. If someone were to ask me what one symptom could be relied upon most, as an indicator that the body has an excess of toxins that must be removed, it would unquestionably be this one. And there is no symptom that has been more grossly misunderstood, much to the astonishment of myself and anyone else familiar with the supreme intelligence and magnificent healing capabilities of the human body. How this most simple and obvious symptom initiated by the wisdom of the body to protect itself has been so outrageously misinterpreted for such a long, long time absolutely boggles the mind. I know you know what I am referring to and have in all likelihood even experienced it at some point in your life. We all have. It's fever.

No matter what your attitude toward fever has been in the past, no matter what you have been led to believe fever is, I want you to know that fever is your friend and ally. I'm not saying that a fever is fun or something you should look forward to, I'm saying that a fever is an activity of the body initiated for the express purpose of protecting itself.

If you were to see a man with blood all over his clothes and on the floor around him, and he just happened to have a butcher knife sticking out of his chest, would there be much doubt in your mind where all the blood was coming from? And what would your reaction be to someone who was supposed to be a medical authority scratching his or her head and saying, "Where in the world is all this blood coming from?" You'd probably look at him or her in the most dumbfounded way possible. Which is exactly how I react every time I hear the standard refrain that fever is one of those deep, dark mysteries that no one has yet been able to figure out. Some of the unfathomable ignorance associated with the explanation and treatment of fevers would make ideal fodder for a comedy routine were the results of that ignorance not so tragic.

Fever patients were *bled!* They were drugged with calomel and quinine, two brutalizing drugs. Fever has always been looked upon as a horror, a demon, a merciless enemy that must be battled and subdued at all cost, even if that meant the death of the patient! This . . . you simply will not believe, but as Mr. Ripley would surely put it, "believe it or not." In the mid-1800s fever patients were denied cool water to drink as it was, of all things, harmful. Children would plead until their throats were too raw to talk, *begging* for water, but it was withheld right up until the patient died. Sometimes when it was thought that the patient was going to die no matter what, the pleading victim was given a glass of water as a dying wish. He or she would miraculously recover, thanks to the water, and *still* the belief was obstinately held on to that water taken cold was "desperate bad for sick folks." A physician of the day who had a more reasonable grasp on reality, once asked to have it explained, "why it was that anything so good for well folks should be so bad for sick folks."[12] How something so inherently beneficial and corrective as a fever, which is initiated by the body to protect itself, has been so horribly misconstrued, is a question for the ages.

A fever mobilizes the body's defenses. When there is an emergency, such as an overaccumulation of toxins in the body, metabolism is accelerated by increasing the amount of heat available, thus enhancing the healing process. This is controlled by the hypothalamus, which is a sort of human thermostat.

Metabolism consists of the absorption of nutrients and the elimination of wastes (toxins). The heat is necessary to accelerate the elimination of toxins which have accumulated beyond the body's ability to tolerate them, and beyond the body's ability to eliminate without some extraordinary modification (i.e., fever). Heat acts as a catalyst which causes the toxins to liquefy and pass into the bloodstream, where they are transported to the organs of elimination (bowels, bladder, lungs, and skin), and thus out of the body.

I still have an article that I clipped out of the newspaper, the headline of which declares, fever still a mystery. The medical doctor offering this bit of dullardism was answering a question from a reader inquiring about what a fever was and what caused it. His answer was, "No one really knows. How fever begins and why it ends is still a mystery."[13] Yeah, it's about as much a mystery as why it's light during daytime and dark during nighttime.

Fever is no mystery. On the contrary, it represents part of the magnificence of the human body, which no scientist or scientists, past or present, have been able to fully comprehend or explain. It is the logical, explainable, totally understandable action of the supremely intelligent human body, merely using one of its numerous mechanisms to protect itself.

And yet, this ignorance around fever persists to this day. I know perfectly intelligent, reasonable people, who are panic-stricken when their child develops a fever. It's off to the doctor for some drugs before the body burns itself up or causes brain damage. The human body is not a stupid lump of clay; it's intelligent beyond our comprehension. The idea that the body would raise its own temperature until there was brain damage is one of the most ridiculous claims I have ever heard.

What do you think the chances are that the body, which is always producing blood, would forget to regulate its production and produce so much blood it drowns in it? What do you think the chances are that the body, after digesting a meal, would forget to stop digesting and digest the stomach? What do you think the chances are that the body, while inhaling and exhaling, all of a sudden forgot to stop inhaling and took in so much air that the lungs exploded? Ridiculous, absurd, outrageous, right? There's no way.

Temperature regulation is one of the most basic and fundamental mechanisms of the human body. It is initiated by the body, controlled by the body, and intelligently and carefully utilized as one of its primary defensive techniques. The very suggestion that this exquisitely designed and managed mechanism of the body would be turned on to accomplish a life-saving function, and then somehow not be turned off until its own brain was fried, is simply foolish. Really! And yet, as recently as late in 1999 we see this medical doctor's comment to a question about fever: "You've hit on a topic that has puzzled the greatest minds of medicine for centuries."[14]

Is it really such a stretch to accept that such a fundamental mechanism as temperature regulation, something the body is involved in *every second of your life,* would be used as a tool to protect and preserve itself? This simple, obvious explanation has confounded the greatest medical minds for centuries. Don't let it confound yours.

In my thirty years of experience, I have never seen or even heard of a single person, young or old, who actually died from a fever, *unless* the fever patient was drugged. A fever is used to facilitate the elimination of toxins. In some instances the burden of a toxic drug with its own inherent side effects, added to the already existing burden of excess toxins in the body, will come together to injure or kill a fever patient. It's the drugs that killed and the fever that was blamed. Do you know what the word "antibiotic" literally means? "Against life"!

Do not fear a fever. Know that it is one of the most common and obvious means by which the body protects itself. If you have a fever, you can be certain that your body is, at the very least, in the second stage of disease or there would be no fever. A patient with a fever should take *no* drugs, eat very, very lightly (ideally fresh fruit and juices exclusively), drink water as desired, stay still, and allow the body to do what it is trying to do without interference. The fever will then accomplish its intended task and subside.

THREE: IRRITATION

Whereas with enervation the only recognizable warning signs are tiredness and loss of appetite, toxemia and its resulting irritation create more recognizable warning symptoms. This stage of disease is designed to make you aware of the rising level of toxins in your body in the hope that you pay attention to the warnings and take the appropriate corrective steps.

Irritation is a condition in which the body sets its defensive mechanisms in motion and speeds up its internal activities in order to unload stored-up toxins. This process can happen at various points in the body. Although irritation is not so painful that it would lead you to visit a doctor for treatment, it is sufficiently unpleasant to make you look for a way to rid yourself of the discomfort. Irritation is the body's way of prodding you into action.

An obvious example of irritation is the urge to urinate or have a bowel movement. This urge is not painful, unless of course it is ignored for a long time, and then it becomes so painful you can think of nothing else but relieving yourself. The bowels and bladder are clearly a most obvious means by which waste and toxins are removed from the body. Less obvious is when toxins are removed at other sites in the body.

Many warning symptoms produced by irritation will be familiar to you. For example, a common warning of irritation due to toxemia is itchiness. The skin is not only the body's largest organ, but also an organ of elimination. The body freely and regularly uses the skin's 4 billion pores to remove toxins from the body, from the top of your head to the bottom of your feet and everything in between. If any part of your skin becomes itchy, that is a classic sign that toxins are being removed; when they reach the surface of the skin, that area becomes irritated. At this stage the condition is not serious or even particularly painful, but it is bothersome, which is the body's way of getting your attention. Only if it is ignored and nothing is done to remove the cause of the problem does the itchiness progress to something far more troublesome. This will be discussed in Stage 4 (inflammation).

Not everyone experiences itchy skin in a state of irritation. Others feel queasy or nauseated for no apparent reason and at different times of day, but particularly in the morning when the body is in its elimination cycle. Another form of irritation is a persistent tickling sensation in the nose. Yet another is to feel jumpy or uneasy or on edge, so that you "fly off the handle" for no apparent reason. If you find yourself uncharacteristically short-tempered or easily aggravated, those are signs of irritation. Certainly you've heard people say things like, "She's so irritable all the time," or "Don't irritate him, he's in a bad mood." People feel irritated because their bodies are in a state of irritation. It's that simple.

Other warning signs of irritation include nervousness, depression, anxiety, and worry, especially when those conditions are out of character for you. You may start to experience more frequent headaches or have minor aches and pains in other areas of your body. Difficulty falling asleep or sleeping fitfully are other indications of irritation. So is putting on weight. Other classic indicators are coated tongue, bad breath, increased body odor, and sallow complexion, especially dark circles under the eyes. Women may experience out-of-the-ordinary menstrual problems or heavier menstrual flow.

You may be thinking, "Good grief, is anything not a warning signal?" That's pretty accurate. Unfortunately, some people live years in a state of irritation without ever knowing what's beating them up. The discomfort they experience isn't serious enough to go for treatment so they just "live with it." But when the effects of enervation, toxemia, and irritation are ignored long enough and the toxic residue that started the whole process in motion builds to an even higher concentration, the fourth stage of disease ultimately, and inevitably, results.

FOUR: INFLAMMATION

Inflammation is the body's most intense effort to cleanse and restore itself. When this process occurs, you become keenly aware that a problem exists, for it involves pain. Pain is not something that occurs haphazardly or without cause. It is not punishment for some indiscretion. *Pain has purpose.*

I told you that this book was going to introduce you to a new way of viewing health and disease. Well, understanding the true nature of pain and the role it plays is a crucial part of that new way of thinking. Pain is your friend. How's that for a new concept? It may not feel comfortable. That's the whole idea. It may not be the friend you would like to have show up on your doorstep, but it is a friend nonetheless. Learning to view pain in a different way will serve you well for the rest of your life. I'm not trying to convince you to like pain; hey, I don't like it any more than you. But I do understand it. And only when you understand it are you going to be able to avoid it.

If you were to accidentally rest your hand on a hot stove, how would you know if it weren't for the pain? If you stepped on a shard of broken glass with your bare foot, how would you know if not for the pain? Pain protects us. It not only warns us that we need to put our hand on something other than a hot stove, but also warns us when our health, our very lives, are at risk. Pain is the body's most effective warning signal. It is specifically designed to alert you to the fact that without corrective measures you are endangering yourself. But because we have not been educated to know this, we fail to recognize that pain is a friendly messenger. When pain is chronic and unrelenting, it is a sign that the body is more desperately attempting to get rid of an ever-increasing level of toxemia before it causes devastating damage. Pain is the means by which the intelligence of the body brings the situation to your attention. Does pain get your attention?

Precious few people realize that pain is a cleansing, healing mode of the body as it tries to fix itself. Instead it is looked upon as an "attack" against your well-being, so it's off to the doctor in search of relief. And sure enough, the doctor will find signs of pathology, which, more often than not, will be treated with drugs. Of course, there will be pathology; after all, that's what the pain is trying to alert us to. The drugs do nothing to *remove* the cause of the problem. They serve only to lessen the pain of the problem. Unfortunately, they are also adding to the body's level of toxemia, while giving the false impression that the problem is being handled. Pain, discomfort, and ill health are the warning signs of what will ultimately cause cells to be driven crazy if not intelligently addressed.

With inflammation, the toxins in the system have usually been concentrated in a particular organ or a particular area of the body for a massive eliminative effort. The area becomes inflamed due to the constant irritation from toxic material. When inflammation exists, we are diagnosed with one or more of the "itises." "Itis" at the end of a word literally means "inflammation of." So tonsillitis means inflammation of the tonsils. Appendicitis—inflammation of the appendix. Hepatitis—inflammation of the liver. Nephritis—inflammation of the kidneys. Arthritis—inflammation of the joints. Colitis—inflammation of the colon. A cold with inflammation of the sinus cavities is rhinitis with sinusitis. The list of "itises" goes on interminably. When a lymph node becomes inflamed, it enlarges and becomes tender. This condition is called "lymphadenitis."[15] A swollen lymph node or gland is one of the body's most obvious warnings that a cleansing of built-up toxins is long overdue. (The lymph system is discussed more fully in the next chapter.)

When irritation of the skin is allowed to progress, it results in dermatitis—inflammation of the skin. Eczema, psoriasis, and a certain type of lupus that affects the skin are particularly severe types of dermatitis and are clear examples of the body using its reparative powers to forcibly push toxins right out through the skin. At this juncture, corrective measures that lower toxic levels in the body will invariably clear up these conditions. I have seen this happen firsthand on numerous occasions.

Sadly, however, people often do not take action at this point. Rather, they suppress the painful symptoms with drugs. The pain may temporarily go away, but the problem doesn't. When the cleansing efforts of the body are suppressed with drugs, the level of toxicity increases until other organs become affected as well, not only with the toxins already in the body but also, as mentioned above, with the added toxicity of the drugs that are administered.

Stage 4 is a pivotal juncture, in that actions taken at this point determine whether or not you are going to recover your health and return to a state of vibrancy, or fall deeper into the diseased state. You are right in the middle of the seven stages and your actions now are crucial. If the body's general toxification is unceasing, it will result in the next stage of disease.

FIVE: ULCERATION

The fifth stage means that the body has been under assault for such a long time that massive amounts of cells and tissue are being destroyed. This condition is often intensely painful because there are exposed nerves. Lesions or ulcers can occur inside or outside the body. An example of an ulcer on the inside is the classic stomach ulcer—a hole in the stomach is literally opened up. Those who have experienced this type of ulcer know all too well how much pain is associated with it. An example of an ulcer on the outside of the body is a canker sore on the mouth, or an open oozing sore on the arm or leg. While the body may use an ulcer as an outlet to rid itself of toxins, it will heal the ulcer if the level of toxemia is sufficiently lowered. Following on the heels of ulceration is the process the body goes through to heal these wounds.

SIX: INDURATION

Scarring is a form of induration, which is a hardening of tissue or the filling in of tissue where it has been lost, such as with an ulcer. But this hardening has real direction and purpose. The toxic material that is threatening the well-being of the body is encapsulated in a sac of hardened tissue. This is the body's way of quarantining the toxic material, holding it in one place so it will not spread freely throughout the body. The sac is a type of tumor and is very often diagnosed as cancer when, in fact, no cancer exists.

Induration is the last stage during which the body is still in control of its cells. If the destructive practices that brought matters to this stage are allowed to continue, cells will start to "go crazy." They will become parasitic, living off whatever nutrients they can obtain, but contributing nothing to the body in return. The constant poisoning has finally altered their genetic encoding and they become wild and disorganized. When cells go wild in this manner, the condition is called cancer.

SEVEN: CANCER

This is the end point in the long evolution of disease, and if the causes that brought it about are continued, it is usually fatal. At this stage, body vitality is at a very low level. Cells are no longer under the control of the brain, but are multiplying wildly in an unorganized manner. Although in the best of circumstances, with a healthy regimen, cancer can be arrested and reversed, it would take a diligent, concentrated effort. The entire purpose of this book is to show you how to prevent this stage from ever occurring.

Contrary to what a staggering number of people think, especially those who have been diagnosed with cancer, your very best friend, your greatest ally in your quest to achieve vibrant health and to prevent cells from being driven crazy, is your body. *Never, ever doubt that.* I cannot tell you how many times I have heard people describe a part of their body as their enemy—as though it were somehow separate and apart and acting on its own. Consider the following statement made by a woman interviewed on a television program on breast cancer aired on PBS. "I had a feeling of wanting very much to get rid of my breasts—they had become my enemies. I wanted to get rid of them, they were something that was going to kill me."[16] Nothing in all of the universe could be further from the truth. Nothing!

People may view the human body as a lot of different parts that are separate from one another, but the body does not see it that way. Every part of the body is as sacred and important and cherished and protected as any other. One organ is just as important and receives just as much healing attention as any other part of the body, be it the breasts, prostate, heart, lungs, teeth, skin, eyes, or intestines. No part receives more or less attention than any other. It's just like when the sun shines, it shines on everything equally. There are no favorites. If something is amiss somewhere in the body, energy is sent to that area in an attempt to correct the problem. And as part of the wisdom inherent in every cell, the body sends messages to us to alert us of any impending problem.

Throughout the first six stages of disease, the body uses discomfort to send us warnings. If the warnings are understood and corrective measures are taken, the warnings stop and the discomfort goes away. If the warnings are not understood and the individual persists in the same habits, the warnings become progressively more acute. The pain continues or becomes more intense. This built-in mechanism is as automatic as the eyes blinking when necessary or blood flowing through the veins. This warning system is yet one more beautiful example of the magnificence of the human body. But all the body can do is warn us to make a change; it can't make the changes for us.

Have you ever been driving down the road and all of a sudden you notice a red light flashing on your dashboard indicating a problem of some sort? What do you do when you see that red light? Do you ignore it in the hope that it will just go away? Do you cover it with tape so you don't have to see it? Or do you take the car into the repair shop as soon as possible to see what the problem is? Car manufacturers have figured out how to put a warning system into automobiles to prevent the destruction of the vehicle. Do you think that God forgot to do the same for us? No! God didn't! No way that God, infinitely wise and intelligent, would forget to give our bodies such a crucially important component as a warning system to protect us from harm.

Keep in mind that health is natural and illness is not. The body always strives to maintain a healthy state. If its health is threatened and warnings appear, it means that the body has not been provided with the best circumstances for maintaining its health and is trying to deal with an overload of toxins. At this point, if corrective action and a healthy lifestyle is adopted, illness will progress no further, the warnings will cease (pain will go away), and health will again return. On the other hand, if the warning signals are suppressed with drugs or ignored, the toxic overload will not be removed. More serious illness will ensue with the final end point being cells driven crazy.

THE DANGER OF DRUGS

Throughout this chapter, I have emphasized that your efforts to take the correct steps to remove the *cause* of any pain or discomfort, rather than silencing those warning signals with drugs, will serve you well for the rest of your life.

Let me now state it plainly: Drugs can be your worst possible enemy. Gulping down drugs at the first sign of discomfort is the old way of thinking, and we are attempting to cultivate a new way of thinking. We have all been conditioned to respond to pain with drugs. It's so easy. You feel pain, you take a drug, the pain goes away, and it's "hurrah for drugs!"

But drugs don't *heal* anything. According to one doctor: "By and large, drugs don't do any good in addressing the underlying causes of illness. Although they can block symptoms that can be life-threatening, in most cases they are overused and misused." Drugs mask symptoms, that's what they're for. Drugs prevent you from doing the right thing for yourself by giving you a false sense of security: "There's no pain so there must be no problem." The problem is hidden, which is why people continue to progress from one stage of disease to the next.

Not surprisingly to me, in 1996 the *Townsend Letter for Doctors,* a leading journal, reported that "The biological action of every prescription drug can essentially be duplicated with nutritional supplements."[17] More and more health-minded doctors are finding that well-chosen, high-quality nutrients and nutraceuticals are able to perform the same task for which a drug was prescribed, but without the harmful side effects that so often accompany prescription drug use. Yet we remain a drugged society. You may recall that I pointed out that we pay a thousand billion dollars a year for health care, and it's projected to be two thousand billion dollars a year by 2007. A lot of that comes from drugs. It's big business. B-I-G business, as Art Buchwald so cleverly underlined in a piece he called "Pill-Pushing for Fun and Profit" with the following line: "Years ago the big profits in the United States were made in oil. These days they come from pharmaceuticals."[18] We consume more than eleven prescription drugs for every man, every woman, and every child in our country.[19] As staggering as that number is, it does not include over-the-counter drugs, which could easily double that number. For natural alternatives to prescription drugs please call 877-335-1509 or go to the web site www.vpnutrition.com.

THE LIVING BODY'S DEFENSE SYSTEM

Dr. Janir Nakouzi

First and foremost, I would like to thank Harvey Diamond for his contribution in helping millions live a healthful lifestyle. Harvey's impact on society has been of tremendous value to many people, including myself.

A good friend of mine asked me to write about the lymphatic system in a way that a lay person could understand. After thinking about how best to do it, I decided to answer the most common questions I was asked by my patients or others who are interested in what I have learned about the subject in my more than thirty years experience with patients and their illnesses.

Why is it important to learn about the lymphatic system? This is one of my patients' most frequently asked questions. Everybody has heard of the "immune system" but not everyone connects it with the lymphatic systems. The most important actions of the immune system occur within or in relationship to the lymphatic system. We all know that our body drains its toxins out by using the liver and kidneys to make stool and urine, but few people know that the lymphatic system acts as a detoxifying organ by draining most of the toxins from the space between the cells, which is called Pischinger's space, intercellular space, matrix, or connective tissue.

What is the lymphatic system and where is it located in the body? My patients say it is easy to understand that the heart is in the middle of the chest and that the liver is a big organ located on the right side of the upper compartment of the abdomen. But when it comes to the lymphatic system, they cannot visualize what it is and where is it located in the body.

That's because the lymphatic system is a *network*, not an organ. In a way, it is very much like the vascular system, the network of blood vessels (arteries and veins) throughout the body. Think of the lymphatic system as a similar network of lymphatic vessels. Like blood vessels, lymphatic vessels are everywhere; there is no area or hidden pocket in the entire human body that the lymphatic system and its vessels do not reach. This system is made of an unbelievably high number, probably somewhere on the order of *trillions* (that is, thousands of billions)—of these tiny lymphatic vessels. There are so many of them everywhere in the body that if you cut yourself, even if it's a minimal cut, you will have severed many of these lymphatic vessels. The smallest lymphatic vessels aggregate into medium-size vessels that then collect into larger vessels, and these finally unite into very large vessels such as the super-size vessel called the *thoracic duct*, which runs in the middle of the chest. The thoracic duct finally drains itself into a large vein that is part of a venous system, called the *superior vena cava*, which goes back inside the heart. Interspersed here and there along the network of smaller lymphatic vessels are centers called *lymph nodes*—much like the service areas on highways. These lymph nodes are in fact service areas for "vehicles" that travel within the lymphatic network like cars on a highway and called *lymphocytes*. "Lympho" refers to the lymphatic system and "cytes" means cells. Just as cars park in a service area in large numbers, the lymphocytes aggregate in the lymph nodes. These aggregates are called *lymphoid tissue* ("tissue" refers to a large number of cells being together for a common purpose or function). This lymphoid tissue is made of cells that have been equipped to perform a specialized function—that is, to defend us from antigens, which are foreign or toxic substances—so they are called *immune competent cells.*

How does the lymphatic system work? Let me illustrate. In every nation there is a police force sent out in each city or territory to look for aberrant behavior. If the body is like a nation, then the organs are the cities, and the tissues are the territories. The body sends out the police force called *antigen presenting cells* or APCs to look for aberrant behavior among citizens of the body (cells) and among foreigners that came into the body (such as viruses, bacteria, or parasites). When the policemen detect something wrong, they report it to the police station for investigation. The police station in the body is the lymph node. Just the way an assigned detective will be sent out from the police station to the crime scene to gather information as part of an investigation, the lymph node sends a T-cell or T-lymphocyte.

The lymph nodes in the body act as detection centers for aberrant behavior. Here's how it works: A police detective gathers information and studies a case, and he will open a file to contain all that information, including everything known about the identity of the suspects (the aberrant cells or harmful foreign substances in the case of the body). He is now the detective officially assigned to the case. In the body the detective who is familiar with the case is called *sensitized immune cell*. Here my illustration reaches its limit, because what the body does with the detective assigned on the case (the sensitized immune cell) cannot be reproduced by a police department: The sensitized immune cell migrates to the lymph node, which in turn produces millions of similar cells that are immune cells sensitized to the same antigens. This migration of the sensitized T-cell from the site of detection to the lymph node is called *homing*. The millions of new cells are called *clones*. Imagine what it would be like if a detective could go to the police station and be cloned to produce millions of other detectives, all of them identical to himself. What actually happens in society is that the detective assigned to the case tries to pass on the information to as many colleagues and policemen as possible to alert them, but these others are never as familiar with the cases as the original detective.

Can we see or feel this homing or cloning? The answer is yes
and no! No, because we are not able to feel or see the homing,
the migration of a single cell, because it is too small for our
senses to detect. But yes, we can feel the cloning part. How?
As the lymph node is forming millions and millions of cells, it
swells, something that we can both see and feel. Did you ever
feel your upper neck when you have a sore throat and discover
that the glands under the angle of your jaw are enlarged?
That's the cloning process taking place. By the way, some parts
of the lymphatic system are so complex and large that we do
not call them lymph nodes but lymph *glands*, such as the sub-
mandibular glands (under the jaw) or the thymus gland (behind
the breast bone). The swelling that we see or feel in these
lymph nodes or glands during an infection is due to the activa-
tion by the sensitized cell of the *immune system cascade*. The
swelling of a lymph node is what we call *inflammation*. The
five descriptive terms referring to inflammation taught to medical students are: *calor, dolor, rubor, tumor,* and *functio laesae*.
Calor is heat or warmth; dolor is pain; rubor is redness; tumor
is the swelling we are speaking about; and functio laesae is the
loss of function. But remember that the inflammation occurring in the lymphatic system is our friend, not our enemy. It is
the mechanism the body puts in place to protect us much the
way the actions taken by the police department (which can
interfere with normal life) are for the protection of the community from harmful elements.

How marvelous this lymphatic system is, capable of activities beyond our unaided comprehension. Thanks to light microscopy and more recently electron microscopy we are able
to explore and understand some of its marvels. This new field
of medical science is called molecular biology. In this field
each lymphocyte becomes as big, relatively speaking, as the
city of New York. New York City is formed of many neighborhoods, such as Little Italy, Chinatown, Soho, and so on.

"Neighborhoods" inside the lymphocyte are called *organelles*, and they have names like nucleus, Golgi apparatus, smooth endoplasmic reticulum, rough endoplasmic reticulum, and many others. The organelles that people may be most familiar with are called *mitochondria* (the energy production engines of lymphocytes). To continue the analogy of city and cell, each neighborhood in New York City is made up of many buildings. Inside the lymphocyte's organelles individual "buildings" are molecules. Some buildings in New York City are very large, such as the Empire State Building, which occupies an entire city block from 33rd to 34th Street. In the cell, these huge buildings are called *macromolecular complexes*. The "Empire State Building" inside the cell would be the *pyruvate dehydrogenase complex*, and it is so enormous that you can see it under the microscope, even though most molecules are not visible.

In this day and age, all of us are bombarded by so much toxicity in the world around us (air, water, food, relationships, homes, lifestyle, the fast pace of living, etc.) that we are loaded with toxins that affect us on all levels, physically, emotionally, mentally, and energetically. We have reached a point where our lymphatic systems are working overtime and around the clock, and becoming depleted. Our lymphatic systems need an initial cleansing to detox them down to a reasonable level, at which we can then maintain them. To accomplish this purpose I created two formulas: Lymphatic Cleanse Formula I and Lymphatic Cleanse Formula II. I formulated them in such a way that anyone, whether young or old, can all benefit from their use. A healthier lymphatic system means a healthier immune system, and a healthier immune system in turn means a better quality of life and increased longevity. That translates into aging more slowly and gracefully.

As one man said, "knowledge is power." Once you have this knowledge about the lymphatic system, you have the power—as well as the responsibility—to do what you know is good for you.

To learn more about cleansing and maintaining a healthy lymphatic system, go to www.drjanirnakouzi.com. You can also ask Dr. Nakouzi your health questions on that site.

FIVE

Your Very Best Friend

I sincerely hope you realize how exquisite you are, how magnificent your body is, what wisdom it possesses. It is capable of performing tasks in such prodigious numbers, and with such perfection, that even to try to comprehend the extent of the intelligence of your body is fruitless. You are a marvel of creation.

There are those in the biological and physiological sciences who are convinced that we will never fully fathom the depth of the intelligence that governs the human body. The brain alone is beyond comprehension. Indeed, the most sophisticated computer ever devised can't compare to the intricacies of the brain. Joined with its other components, your body is unmatched in power, capacity, and adaptability.

As you learned earlier, the human body comprises 100 trillion cells, all working in perfect harmony. Each organ is a marvel in itself. The heart pumping 6 quarts of blood through 96,000 miles of blood vessels. The digestive tract turning food into flesh and blood. Balance always being maintained, temperature always being kept stable. Lungs supplying oxygen to the cells. More than 200 bones and more than 600 muscles working together to enable you to move in any direction anytime you wish. Ears that allow you to enjoy music. Eyes to behold the glories of a sunset. A sense of smell to marvel at the scent of a rose. Taste buds to take pleasure from food. And more activities, too numerous to list, all proceeding with extraordinary precision, simultaneously, for a hundred years or more, if need be. It is staggering to try to grasp the infinite intelligence necessary to coordinate the activities and precision of the human body. We can only stand in humble awe of it.

THE MAGNIFICENT HUMAN BODY

There is a force, an energy, that resides in each of us that directs and governs all the functions described above and more. That energy was what transformed you from an infinitesimal bit of protoplasm into the astonishing being you are today. It is that energy that "knows" instantly what to do if you cut your finger. Without any conscious action on your part, the blood coagulates, a scab forms, the wound seals itself, the scab falls off, and presto, no more cut. What heals a broken bone after a fracture? Is it the cast and sling? Of course not. It is the wisdom and power of the body that heals. A substance more powerful than any glue is secreted by the bone at both points of fracture, and the two segments are reunited as strongly or stronger than before the break. This process is neither chemical nor physical (i.e., man-made). It is biological! Even if you were to fall and break several bones and sustain several cuts, all of them would be healed simultaneously, while all the other myriad functions of the body were also being performed. Such is the power inherent in the energy that directs the activities of the human body.

This energy, this force that has been with you since the beginning of your life, never leaves you as long as you are alive. It is an integral part of your existence. This energy that miraculously heals wounds is always there to carry out other, even more serious healing. From this point on, you can be totally confident that whether you are in a state of exuberant health or failing health, this energy is automatically striving for your highest possible level of health under all circumstances. It can do nothing else, as this is why it exists! It is with you fully at this very moment and always will be. My goal is to create in you a sense of reverence for this powerful energy, reverence that will lead you to support your body in its ability and effort to provide you with vibrant health.

We should be in a constant state of astonishment over our bodies, yet we take them largely for granted. We must nurture a genuine appreciation for the unparalleled ability to heal that our bodies possess.

It is precisely in this area of acknowledgment of the appreciation for the remarkable power of the body to protect and heal itself that the "experts" have somehow managed to commit the most astonishing oversight in all the history of the healing professions. What is so mind-boggling is that what they have missed is so glaringly obvious that there's really no accounting for why it has been missed. It's just one of those unexplained mysteries.

THE LYMPH SYSTEM: THE BODY'S GARBAGE COLLECTOR

I wonder if you happen to have a recollection similar to one I have that goes something like this: As a youngster I was asked by my mother to get the butter from the refrigerator and bring it to the dinner table. "Sure, Mom," I said as I jumped up from the table and headed for the fridge. After opening the refrigerator door, the following conversation ensued between me in the kitchen and my mother in the dining room:

"It's not here, Mom."

"It certainly is, I put it there myself."

"I'm looking all over. It's not here."

"Open your eyes. It's right in the front."

"I'm tellin' you, Mom, my eyes are open. It's not here!"

"Don't make me come in there and get it myself."

"Mom! Somebody must have taken it already."

At this point she strode into the kitchen, walked up to me and the open refrigerator, and without so much as a glance, reached in and picked up the butter dish, which was on the middle shelf *right in front!* I couldn't believe I was looking right at it and didn't see it. If it were any closer to me, it would have stained my shirt.*

What the authorities have missed should have been as obvious to them as the butter dish should have been to me. The only difference is that my oversight has not resulted in the unnecessary loss of life.

By now you must be asking, "My God, what is it? What did they miss?" Only the single most important factor in the prevention not only of disease, but also of the years of pain and ill health that lead up to it. It falls under the category of "the dynamics of the human body." Herein lies the most fundamental difference between the standard medical approach and that of Natural Hygiene. Hygiene looks at the human body as dynamic and capable, always aware of problems that may exist and constantly on top of dealing with them. Traditional medicine looks at the human body as a hapless victim, forever at the mercy of any and all malevolent beasts that may attack it.

Specifically, I am talking about the body's lymph system. This magnificent system's purpose has long been misunderstood and its activities misinterpreted. As part of the incredible intelligence of the human body, there are several systems that

---

*I don't think I'll ever forget the look on my mom's face when she picked up that butter dish. She gave me the kind of look that was a cross between annoyance and disgust that she might give if she were to see someone pick his nose and wipe it on his sleeve.

perform seemingly miraculous functions: the nervous system, cardiovascular system, respiratory system, digestive system, reproductive system, musculoskeletal system, and lymph system which is an integral part of the body's defense system.

Your body is infinitely capable of defending and protecting itself. Our creator thought of absolutely *everything* when making our bodies. God didn't forget something as critically important and essential as a mechanism to protect against disease. That is the defense system, erroneously referred to as the "immune system." There is no such thing as an "immune system." It would be lovely if we could be made "immune," but it doesn't work that way. And you may think I am merely splitting hairs by calling it the "defense system" rather than the "immune system." Not so.

If you hold a loaded gun to your head and pull the trigger, there is no immunity to blowing your brains out. And there is no immunity to violating the laws of nature for years on end and not having to pay the price for doing so. People have been convinced that they can live an unhealthy lifestyle, then run to the doctor for a pill or shot that will make everything okay, as if miraculously, all past transgressions can be swept away by some potion. That's delusionary thinking that ultimately leads to one's demise. So throughout the book, whenever I refer to what is traditionally called the "immune system," I will be calling it the defense system.

As far as preventing disease and creating vibrant health are concerned, your success depends on understanding the lymph system, which is the heart and soul of the body's defense mechanism. The lymph system is not at all complicated. You already know something of it. Most of what you know about the "immune system" is actually the work of the lymph system.

As discussed in Chapter Four, toxins are a major contributing factor in the development of disease. There is just no getting around this fact. No understanding of disease will ever be reached if the role played by toxemia and the lymph system is not also understood.

If toxins are allowed to build up and remain in the body, they will eventually cause harm to some degree, anything from general aches and pains all the way to driving cells crazy. If, however, they are removed from the body on a regular basis so that what is being built up is not allowed to exceed what is eliminated, your system will be kept sufficiently clean to prevent disease from ever getting started. Does it not, therefore, make all the sense in the world to do whatever you possibly can to assist and facilitate the mechanism in your body responsible for removing toxins?

How fortunate we are that our bodies are equipped with such supreme intelligence. You may not have ever thought specifically about it before, but isn't it absolutely amazing that your body knows how to turn an apple into blood? It's really quite a remarkable feat if you think about it. In this technologically advanced world, there is no scientist anywhere on earth who can go into a laboratory and turn food into blood. Yet the body accomplishes this formidable task as a matter of course right along with all the other equally impressive feats it performs.

It is with the same intelligence, ability, and precision that the body performs all its functions, including the removal of toxins from the body. Enter the lymph system.

Do you remember a few years back when the New York City Department of Sanitation went on strike and refused to pick up any garbage? I don't recall how long the strike lasted, but I do know it was long enough to become an abominable situation for New Yorkers. The mere sight of huge piles of garbage everywhere you looked was depressing enough, but such a prodigious amount of garbage accumulated that it actually blocked sidewalks for pedestrians and, in some instances, spilled out into the streets, impeding traffic. Worse yet was the stench, horrendous enough to take the enamel off your teeth.

Every day the evening news brought us pictures of the ever-worsening crisis and the comments of frustrated and disgusted New Yorkers. It was, in no uncertain terms, a great big ugly, stinking mess that, if not corrected, would have eventually shut down the city. Guess what I'm getting at? The lymph system is, quite literally, your body's garbage collector. Although it can be overwhelmed, fortunately for us, our garbage collector never goes on strike. It is hard at work twenty-four hours a day in its relentless effort to keep the inside of the body cleansed and rejuvenated.

I hope I have succeeded in giving you a sense of the magnificence of your body, of the incomprehensible wisdom by which it is governed. You can be totally confident that the incomparable intelligence with which the lymph system carries out its many functions is no exception.

The lymph system is an astounding network of fluid, organs, nodes and nodules, ducts, glands, and vessels that continuously and aggressively cleanse the system of waste matter. Millions upon millions of nodes, some minuscule, some large, guard the passages into the body against the intrusion of destructive substances. Placed end to end in a straight line, all the lymph vessels in the body would cover a distance in excess of 100,000 miles. They would circle the globe four times![35] There is three times as much lymph fluid in your body as there is blood.[36] That should tell you something of its importance.

Unlike the circulatory blood system, the lymph system carries fluid only *away* from the tissues. It picks up wastes from all the cells and, through an intricate series of processes, breaks them down and arranges for their elimination from the body. The lymph system is also involved in the production of white blood cells (lymphocytes) that seek out, capture, and destroy foreign substances such as bacteria and other "invaders," and remove them from the body as well.

The circulation of lymph provides ample opportunity for toxins to come in contact with the surfaces of the body's powerful cleansing cells, such as macrophages and lymphocytes. More than 99 percent of soluble toxins (called antigens) can be trapped in the body's lymph nodes.[37]

PHYSIOLOGY OF THE LYMPH SYSTEM

Except for cartilage, nails, and hair, your entire body is bathed in lymph. If you could somehow see a picture of the network of glands and nodes inside your body, you would see what looked like an extremely fine sheath of lace covering and saturating everything. You can actually feel some lymph nodes where they are close to the surface of your skin. You can most easily feel lymph nodes on the sides of your neck, under your chin, under your arms, and where your legs meet your torso.

If you would like to see some unusually large lymph nodules, open your mouth and look at your tonsils. This, of course, will not be possible for a huge segment of the population, because before it was realized how extremely important and beneficial the tonsils were, they were removed willy-nilly as though they were some mistake of nature. Now that it is known that the tonsils are an integral part of the lymph system, forming a protective ring of lymph tissue around the opening between the nasal and oral cavities that provides protection against bacteria and other potentially harmful materials,[38] they are allowed to stay where God put them.

The traditional attitude that the tonsils are expendable demonstrates how this marvel of creation—the lymph system—has not been given the understanding and respect it deserves. Indeed, it has been entirely overlooked as the protector of our health.

I remember traveling through London in 1988, and while reading the local newspaper there, I saw an article with the headline TONSILS BARGAIN. Evidently, in an effort to facilitate the removal of these troublesome and obviously useless organs, physicians gave their time free and set up an assembly line so that over two weekends children could have their tonsils removed at a very low cost. According to the head of the health department who arranged the Tonsil Bargain: "We did 128 operations last Easter and it was such a success we thought we would repeat the exercise."[39] I had my tonsils summarily removed at age three. In those days (late 1940s), having them taken out was almost automatic. Tonsils were considered a kind of practical joke that God stuck in our throats. They were an affliction. The attitude to their removal was good riddance. Tragic, really.

When the tonsils enlarge, swallowing becomes very uncomfortable. It's almost as though the body is trying to tell us, "Hey, stop eating for a while so I can catch up and clear things out." And instead of being educated to understand the message our tonsils are sending us and taking the appropriate action, we tear them out at the roots and get a big bowl of ice cream as a reward for being cooperative while they were being removed.

You do not need an in-depth, highly technical understanding of all the physiological functions of the lymph system. In fact, for the purposes of preventing ill health in general, and disease in particular, you know practically all you need to know about it. The main thing is to know that toxins build up in your body. If they are not removed, they will cause you pain, make you sick, and eventually drive certain cells crazy, making them cancer cells, and that is the explicit function of the infinitely capable lymph system: to break down and remove toxins from the body before they can cause harm.

I think the best way to inform you about the lymph system and how it does its impressive work is to give you an example to relate to. I've decided to use breast cancer as the example and let me tell you why. First of all, it seems to be in the news all the time, and the next chapter happens to deal with breast cancer specifically. Second, it helps me to solidify in your mind what I expressed earlier, which is that cancer is cancer no matter where in the body it occurs or what name it is given. I could have just as easily said I would use prostate cancer, colon cancer, or any other. Remember, where in the body cells are driven crazy is of no importance. That some cells in the body were finally driven crazy as the result of continued neglect and abuse is what is of importance. And since lymph nodes and the lymph system are always involved in cancer no matter where in the body it appears, and whenever the subject of breast cancer arises, there is invariably mention made of lymph nodes and the lymph system, it seemed the perfect example.

Now, don't forget, the word "cancer" is just that, a word. We can attach any meaning to it we wish. We can see it as a horror that descends like a plague, or as something totally understandable and avoidable. For the purposes of this book and your effort to know how to have complete and total control over whether or not you live in health or ill health, you have to think of the word "cancer" as something other than what you may have thought it was all your life. You mustn't think of it as something that can somehow sneak itself into the body and do harm, but rather the result of using drugs to suppress the warning signals from the body for years on end as the disease state progressed from stage to stage until the body could no longer protect its cells from harm.

There is no more obvious evidence that the body is struggling to remove toxins than finding a lump (swollen lymph node) somewhere in the body, because that lump is swollen with toxins that the body has cordoned off to prevent them from circulating through the system, causing harm.

There's nothing to fear from finding a lump somewhere in your body because it is the nature of the lymph system that you have had many lumps (swollen lymph nodes) come and go without your ever being slightly aware of them. So there's no need to panic if you find one. You should actually be grateful that your body has the intelligence and ability to use its lymph nodes to hold the toxins in check until you take the proper steps to empty them from the nodes and eliminate them from the body. This is, of course the purpose of the CARE principles.

Lymph nodes fill up and empty all the time; the frequency with which this happens depends upon the level of toxemia in your body and the amount of vital energy your body has to empty them. That is why Dr. Susan Love says, "If you feel a lump the first thing you should do is take a deep breath. There is no rush. Even the diagnosis of cancer is not an emergency. And certainly the diagnosis of a lump is not an emergency. There are twelve benign lumps for every cancer."[40]

I find it criminal that women have been whipped into such a frenzy of fear over searching out and finding lumps in their breasts. Women have actually been taught to fear the normal activities of their bodies rather than to understand and appreciate them. We fear the unknown. Once you know what the lumps are, however, why they have appeared, and how simply you can facilitate their removal, fear will no longer have a hold over you. This, of course, is true not only for swollen lymph glands in a woman's breast, but also for lumps and swollen glands anywhere in the body.

As I am a devoted fan of the analogy as a learning tool, I will use one here to explain a few things about lumps and lymph nodes. Think of a fountain that has water forced up its center. When the water reaches the top, it cascades onto a series of shallow, bowl-shaped ledges. The fountain is like a Christmas tree in shape in that the top ledge is small and all the ledges below increase in diameter. As the water fills the top bowl-like ledge, it spills over into the next ledge below it. As that ledge fills, water spills over into the larger one below it and so on until all the ledges are filled and the last one at the bottom spills over into the pool and a pump sends the water back up the center of the fountain. I've seen miniature versions of this type of decorative fountain at parties, used to dispense fruit punch. To fill your glass, you simply hold it under one of the ledges where the punch is overflowing. It is a simplistic comparison, perhaps, but the activities of the lymph system with its network of lymph nodes work similarly to that of the fountain: The waste matter in your body is the water and the lymph nodes are the ledges that fill and overflow.

Now remember, waste matter—toxins—are constantly being produced and built up, picked up by the lymph system, and removed from the body. Lymph nodes are truly amazing little processing plants. As an indispensable component of the body's defense system, lymph nodes filter out bacteria and other foreign material from lymph fluid which constantly flows through the nodes. This waste material is broken down, degraded, and sent on its way for elimination. When the level of waste in the body builds at a greater pace than it is eliminated, the lymph nodes are overburdened and they enlarge. They simply cannot keep up. As lymph nodes swell and fill to capacity, the waste moves on to the next available node. Frequently, these swollen lymph nodes are surgically removed, especially if cancerous cells are detected in them. But removing the nodes is not removing the problem. The problem is the ever-increasing level of toxic waste, not the nodes that are trying to contain it.

Let's return to the fountain analogy for a moment. Do you think for one fleeting moment that removing one of the ledges near the top of the fountain that is filling with water would prevent the water from getting to the other ledges? Even the removal of all the ledges would not impede the water's progress one iota. The only way to prevent the ledges from filling with water is not to remove them, but to stem the flow of water. So, the only way to prevent lymph nodes from enlarging is not to remove them, but to stem the flow of wastes flowing into them. Imagine the dire consequences of removing all the lymph nodes in the body because they'd become enlarged. The defense system would be so severely impaired that premature death would inevitably follow as poisons flowed freely through the "undefended" body. Your body is your citadel of life. Your lymph nodes are your warriors, your guardians, performing an indispensable service protecting you from harm. You can't live without them!

ROAD TO THE TRUTH

There is something I wish to share with you. During the writing of this book, whenever I needed some bit of information or some help, as though by divine grace, I got exactly what I needed when I needed it. What I needed came to me in totally unexpected ways so many times that I simply can't help thinking that it was more than mere coincidence. If I needed a certain piece of information, it would show up in the mail, in an article sent to me by someone who thought for some reason I would be interested in it. Or I needed a certain lead and I would see what I was looking for on the cover of a magazine in a bookstore.

The very day that I was ruminating on whether these were coincidences or divine intervention, a friend told me about a book that she thought I would enjoy, *The Celestine Prophecy* by James Redfield. I wasn't doing a lot of reading outside of the subject I was working on, but I picked up the book to take a look at it because I was beginning to get the hint that these "coincidences" weren't coincidences. The book describes nine key insights into life that will help readers experience a deeper spiritual awareness. The first of the insights describes how everything happens in life on schedule, with purpose—that there are no coincidences. You could have knocked me over with a feather.

I knew from the very beginning of this project that this particular chapter was going to be one of the most important and pivotal chapters in the book. First, it explains what lumps in the body are, and the incredible lymph system that is behind them, which is crucial to your understanding how the three principles of CARE (see Part II) will help you prevent disease and achieve vibrant health. Second, it is no small matter to state that the experts in charge have somehow missed something as significant as the lymph system's role in preventing disease rather than being victimized by it.

The proof of that evidence is the frequency with which lymph nodes are routinely removed from a woman's chest, side, and arms as a treatment for breast cancer, and how little provocation is needed for this procedure. I know many women whose physicians convinced them to allow the removal of lymph nodes from under their arms as a "safety measure." That would be like tearing out your alarm system at home as a safety measure against burglary.

Anyway, one day I was at my desk working on this chapter and I received a phone call from a friend to whom I had not spoken for some time and who lives far away. After I told him about my project, he mentioned, almost as an afterthought, that he'd been looking through a really first-rate book, *Anatomy and Physiology,* which was used as a textbook and was beautifully written and illustrated. He said he remembered reading some interesting material on the lymph system. After all the similar experiences I'd had, I recognized his call and the book he mentioned as another of these "coincidences." Because it was an academic book, it was not available in any bookstore in my town. But I found a store in the state willing to FedEx it to me.

I received the book the next day, and I immediately sat down and read the chapter entitled "Lymphatic Organs and Immunity." Have you ever been watching a movie, a taut suspense-thriller in which someone is trying to find some lost or hidden piece of evidence to solve a mystery? After following numerous leads, that elusive piece of evidence is finally found. The suspense has built to a nerve-wracking crescendo, and at the moment when the hero finds what he's been looking for, the camera moves in for a close-up on his face, a fanfare sounds, and the person who has been searching so long and hard pumps a clenched fist in the air and yells, *"Yes!"* I came to a passage in that chapter on the lymph system that made me feel that same surge of excitement, and I looked around for the movie camera, fully expecting to hear the fanfare. At that moment, I would not have been the least bit surprised if Steven

Spielberg himself stood up behind me and said, "Cut! That's a wrap!" The short, simple passage spoke volumes. At first I couldn't believe my eyes, so I read it over carefully again and again. It was as if all my work and effort had been rewarded with one simple sentence found in the last place on earth I would expect, or even hope, to find it: in a medical textbook.

The passage reads:

> Cancer cells can spread from a tumor site to other areas of the body through the lymphatic system. At first, however, as the cancer cells pass through the lymph system, they are trapped in the lymph nodes, which filter the lymph. During cancer surgery, malignant (cancerous) lymph nodes are often removed, and their vessels are cut and tied off to prevent the spread of the cancer.[41]

So what is so momentous about this? You may well ask. Let me highlight the sentence that jumped off the page at me like a pit bull going after a steak, and explain why it is of such significance:

> At first, however, as the cancer cells pass through the lymph system, *they are trapped in the lymph nodes,* which filter the lymph.

This sentence confirms what I have been stating. How? It shows that although traditional medicine may have a masterful understanding of the *technical* functions of the lymph system, there is no understanding of the *practical* functions it performs. Whereas Natural Hygiene sees the body as dynamic, as the actor, traditional medicine sees the body as passive, as a victim. Thus we so often hear about how cancer spreads and works itself into a lymph node, requiring the node's removal. But it is made very clear in that passage from the textbook that cancer cells don't work their way into a lymph node, the cancer cells are "trapped by" the lymph nodes.

Indeed, a cancer cell works its way into a lymph node in the same way a piece of dirt "works its way" into a vacuum cleaner. The lymph node is doing something to the cancer cells. It's not the other way around! No wonder "they don't know." They have reversed the entire order of things. (Talk about not seeing the butter in the refrigerator, how about not even seeing the refrigerator in the kitchen?) It is similar to when the earth was believed to be fixed in space with the sun circling it, because the sun could be seen moving across the sky. Of course, now we know that it only *looks* as if the sun is moving; in fact, it isn't. It only looks as if cancer cells are attacking lymph nodes; in fact, they aren't.

As cancer cells are carried by the lymph fluid, they are brought to lymph nodes, where they are trapped. Let's look at this more closely. I have made the point over and over how magnificently intelligent the human body is. It "knows" what it's doing. It performs trillions of actions and reactions; no activity is wasted, none are superfluous, all have an absolute reason for taking place. The body has far too much to do to busy itself with activities that don't directly contribute to its own survival. So you can be sure beyond even a shadow of a doubt that if the body traps cancer cells in its lymph nodes, it has a damn good reason for doing so!

The lymph nodes contain phagocytic cells. *Phago* means eat and *cytic* means cell. Eating cells gobble up and degrade foreign substances. Cancer cells are trapped there as the body's last line of defense. Remember, cancer is the seventh and last stage of disease. During the first six stages when cancer could have been prevented by certain lifestyle changes but wasn't, the next stage kept inevitably following the previous one until cells were driven crazy. As a last-ditch effort to deal with the cancer cells that have obviously broken away from their original site and started to spread through the lymph system, the body traps them in the lymph nodes.[42]

There is no other possible reason that the body would make this effort. The body never gives up the fight no matter how bad things are, no matter how serious the situation, no matter how ongoing the neglect. As long as it is alive, the body strives for homeostasis—for balance. Like water in a jar that seeks its own level no matter what position the jar is in, the body seeks to normalize, correct, and maintain balance no matter what the circumstances. Even in the face of such long-standing abuse and neglect that cells are driven crazy, the body still has the wherewithal to call to arms its last sentinels guarding the health of the body: those amazing, cancer-trapping, protective lymph nodes.

And how are these precious lymph nodes treated? They are cut out! And why? For performing the very function they were created and intended to perform!

Nothing, and I mean nothing, could be more backward. Would you allow your bladder to be cut out because of the presence of urine? Would you allow your colon to be cut out because of the presence of feces? Would you allow your lungs to be cut out because of the presence of carbon dioxide? Can you imagine a more preposterous suggestion than that? The removal of one of your vital organs for doing the very job it was put there to do? It is every bit as preposterous to remove a lymph node for doing its job as it is to remove the bladder, colon, or lungs for doing their job.

We look back in amazement and disbelief that our ancestors were so blind to the dynamics of the body that they routinely drained blood from the sick. Bleeding patients was a standard, universally accepted practice. It was believed that as the blood ran out of the body, so would the sickness. Removing lymph nodes for doing the job they were created to do, at the very moment when what they are doing is most needed—preventing the wild, uncontrolled spread of cancer cells—makes bleeding look like the cornerstone of scientific wisdom.

And just where, pray tell, will the waste and cancer cells go when these lymph nodes are removed? To the next available lymph nodes, that's where. Removing one of the ledges in the fountain won't stop the water from going to the next available ledge, and removing a bunch of lymph nodes won't stop the cancer from going to the next available node. That's why it is so common to hear, "You've relapsed," or "We didn't get it all." Because until the buildup and flow of wastes and toxins in the body are curtailed, you can excise every lymph node in the body and it will be to no avail. That is because the swollen lymph node is only the symptom of a cause that is not being addressed. Under those conditions, "relapse" is inevitable.

I must say I was enormously encouraged in late 1996 when I read an article published in the journal *Surgical Oncology Clinics of North America* that said, "Lymph node removal in an increasing number of breast cancer cases is done as a matter of tradition and history, not medical necessity." Some women, the authors said, "are needlessly enduring a lifetime of swollen or numb arms and a high risk of infection because doctors have been indiscriminate about removing lymph nodes." This is because, "It was once thought that cancer from the lymph nodes could be spread to other organs or tissue through the lymph fluid. It has since been proved that the lymph nodes don't spread cancer—they merely tell doctors if the cancer has already spread." They went so far as to state that, "Even with some invasive cancers—it might be possible, or even advisable, to forgo lymph node removal." That change could, they suggest, "spare many women from the disabling side effects of lymph node removal." I was pleased that the authors stated, "One should have the courage not to do lymph node removal as a routine."[43] As encouraging as all this is, there is still a long way to go before there is a full understanding of the lymph system.

When O.J. Simpson was in custody awaiting trial, he had a lymph node removed from under his arm to determine if it was cancerous. It turned out that it wasn't. The attending physician diagnosed the swollen lymph node as "benign reactive lymphocytic hyperplasia." Translated into English, that is the abnormal growth of normal white blood cells that results in the increased size of the node.

Now, even the most elemental understanding of the role lymph nodes play in the lymph system's job of keeping the body clean tells us what was happening in this case. The body increased production of white blood cells to deal with an overload of toxins in the body that had started to accumulate in the lymph nodes. It's the body's defense system in action. Simple. Obvious. Elemental. But the media stated that "further studies" were going to be conducted to try to "determine the cause of the swelling" of the node.[44] Studies? That would be like pulling a floundering person out of a swimming pool and then doing "further studies" to determine why the person was soaking wet.

POISONED BACK TO HEALTH?

I was deeply saddened by the passing of Jacqueline Kennedy Onassis. Not so much because she was the widow of one of the presidents of the United States or that she was a woman of great courage, style, and dignity who had gone through so much in her private and public life. I was saddened by the fact that she became yet one more victim in a long and heartrending line of victims to lose their lives because of a lack of understanding of the basic needs of the human body. History will record that Jacqueline Kennedy Onassis died of cancer. And most assuredly cells had been driven crazy in her body. But I believe that ignorance of the dynamics of her lymph system hastened her death.

There is a simple, logical, commonsense axiom in Natural Hygiene. It is so obvious that one might think it is ludicrous even to mention. Here it is: You cannot be poisoned back to health. Does that seem reasonable to you? But lo and behold there is also a medical axiom. Remember, I mentioned it earlier? In Latin it is *Ubi virus, ibi virtus.* Translation: Where there is poison, there is virtue. If you were in a bookstore, would you be sufficiently interested to spend your money on a book entitled *How to Poison Yourself Back to Health*? Probably every fiber of your being would revolt against such a suggestion; yet medical treatment dictates that those who are sickest be poisoned the most.

Radiation and chemotherapy are poisons. They poison and kill both cancer cells and healthy cells. Moreover, these treatments are themselves carcinogenic. That's right, the treatment for cancer *causes* cancer. Back in the early eighties, health-care workers who were involved with the preparation and administration of anticancer drugs were warned to take special precautions when handling the drugs because of the risk of developing cancer from being in contact with them. An article published by the American Cancer Society states that the increased risk "should be of great concern to those handling anticancer agents."[45]

So, those *handling* the drugs should be greatly concerned. What about the people having them injected directly into their veins! No need for concern there? If a strong, healthy, fit, and vibrant person were to be given intense radiation and chemotherapy, that individual would quickly become debilitated, devitalized, and sick. How then could the same treatment given to someone who is already sick be expected to make that person well? Where's the common sense? If something will make a well person sick, it will surely make a sick person sicker. How could it possibly be otherwise?

As I read articles describing the cancer treatment given to Mrs. Onassis, I was filled with sorrow and dread. In the midst of the assault she was under, I commented to a friend that Mrs. Onassis couldn't possibly live out the week. She died the next day.

Mrs. Onassis had lymphoma. "Oma" means tumor, so what she had was a tumor in her lymph system, meaning one or more of her lymph nodes were found to have cancer cells in them. *Trapped there,* no doubt, by her body as it struggled as best it could with the results of years of toxemia within her system. Had the affected lymph nodes been in her breasts, she would have been told that she had breast cancer. If cancer is diagnosed in a lymph node, it is described as a lymphoma (i.e., non-Hodgkin's lymphoma). In fact, a tumorous lymph node in the breast could be called lymphoma as well.

Newspaper accounts of Mrs. Onassis's cancer and treatment said that her cancer "attacked" the lymph system and that "tumors can arise anywhere there are lymph nodes and lym- phatic channels." She became acutely aware of her problem when in December 1993 she "noted a swelling in her right groin." A physician diagnosed a swollen lymph node. A few weeks later she developed a "cough, swollen lymph nodes in her neck and pain in her abdomen." She was examined and her doctor found "enlarged lymph nodes in her neck and in her armpit." A CAT scan (a computerized X ray) showed that "there were swollen lymph nodes in her chest and in an area deep in her abdomen."[46]

To a Natural Hygienist, in tune with the dynamics of the body and the knowledge of the important role the lymph system plays, these signals could not have been clearer. Mrs. Onassis needed to allow her system to be cleansed of toxins and waste and she needed it fast.

Instead of realizing that cancer cells had been trapped in lymph nodes as an attempt to cordon them off from the rest of the body until they could be dealt with, traditional medicine looked upon them as helpless victims under attack by maraud- ing cancer cells. In response to that view, a course of very aggressive radiation and chemotherapy was undertaken and the former first lady's fate was sealed. She was bombarded with drugs. Lots of powerful, virulent, energy-sapping, life- diminishing drugs. The *New York Times* stated that she "ini- tially responded to therapy, but it [cancer] came back in her brain and spread through her body."[47]

For the unrelenting pain in her neck, Mrs. Onassis received more drugs. For the acute pneumonia she developed in her weakened state, she received more drugs. Steroids were part of the mixture in her chemotherapy, which caused a perforated ulcer in her stomach. In the middle of her ordeal, she had to be operated on to sew up the hole in her stomach. She went from bad to worse, and as a final assault on her body, she was subjected to even more radiation and chemotherapy, only this time it was shot directly into her brain. The cancer spread to her spinal cord, her liver, and throughout her body. She became weak and disoriented, lost weight, developed shaking chills, her speech slowed, and she had difficulty walking.

How Mrs. Onassis held on for as long as she did under such a barrage of poisonous chemicals is a testament to her strength and will to live. The fact is, her body was already weak from her own internal struggle to deal with the cancer in her lymph system. Add to that a relentless attack with the most virulent poisons on earth and she didn't stand an ice cube's chance in the sun. After it was apparent that all hope of recovery was gone, the headline in the *New York Times* read: DOCTORS TOLD MRS. ONASSIS THAT THERE WAS NOTHING MORE THEY COULD DO. I'd say!

There's a very good reason why, when oncologists, doctors who specialize in the treatment of cancer, were asked if they would opt for chemotherapy if they or their loved ones were ever diagnosed with cancer, 75 percent said no. How ironic that the constant contact with toxins—poisons—is what drives cells crazy in the first place and it is *more* poisons that are then used to try to destroy those cells. It is the elements of health, not poisons, that will produce good health, recapture it if it is lost, and maintain it once found.

I watched the same scenario unfold in 1963 when my father was only fifty-seven years old. He'd been diagnosed with cancer. It was bad, but nothing compared to the aftermath of the radiation and chemotherapy he endured. I was only eighteen at the time and had not yet learned what I know now, so obviously I couldn't exert any influence on the decisions being made on his behalf. He is one reason that my life's work is to help people avoid a fate similar to his.

A few days after Mrs. Onassis's death, there was an article in the *New York Times* with a headline that made me shake my head in exasperation. It read: LYMPHOMAS ARE ON THE RISE IN U.S., AND NO ONE KNOWS WHY."[48] In the article, there were statements like, "No one knows precisely why." "Experts are stymied." "Doctors know little." "Reasons are poorly understood." It always amazes me that whenever medical scientists don't know something, they immediately declare that "no one knows." It's not true.

Sure enough, five years later in 1999, an article appeared on the drop in lung cancer due to a decline in smoking. It noted, however, that other cancers are not faring so well, and it stated, "New cases of non-Hodgkin's lymphoma are rising by 1.8 percent a year." That was followed by the old refrain: "No one knows why."[49] Well, my friend, I know why. And now, you do as well.

I am very fortunate to have several friends who are doctors who are not threatened by the fact that although I am not medically trained, I can sufficiently challenge their thinking on certain aspects of traditional medical treatment to make them stop and reflect. One of these friends, whom I have known for more than a dozen years and with whom I am very close, asked me what approach I was going to take in telling people how to prevent cells from being driven crazy. I told him my approach focuses on an understanding of the lymph system, how it works and how to keep it sufficiently clean so as to prevent tumors from appearing. After explaining to him the Natural Hygiene view of how the lymph system operates, I asked him point-blank, "How is it that medical doctors, including you, can go to school for twelve years and come away with no understanding of the crucial role the lymph system plays in preventing disease?" He thought for a few moments and said, "You know what, Harvey? I don't know why. It's just not stressed. We learn the mechanics of it, but not its practical application." And it is this epic oversight that is the very reason that so many of the experts "don't know" how to prevent cells from being driven crazy.

Here is my message to you, dear reader: Don't worry! By applying the principles of CARE (see Part II), you will know how to deal with cancer, because by understanding and respecting the activities and needs of your lymph system, you will be taking the appropriate steps to prevent it from ever occurring in the first place.

SIX

Keeping Abreast

Excuse me, sir? Were you about to skip over this chapter because you have no interest in breast cancer? If it were about prostate cancer, would that rekindle your interest? If so, then read on, because that *is* what it's about. I know I will be running the risk of repeating myself to the point that you might call out, "All right already!" However, brand-new concepts frequently have to be repeated for the very reason that they are new information. And I would much prefer to say something too much than not enough.

So, here goes. There is no difference between breast cancer and prostate cancer except for the fact that one occurs in a man's body, and one occurs primarily in a woman's body. Other than that, they are the exact same phenomenon, simply appearing at different locations. If you took your car out of your garage and left it in the parking lot at the store, it's still a car, isn't it? It's not called a truck or a bus only because it's somewhere other than in your garage.

With sufficient neglect over a long enough time, cells can be driven crazy—anywhere in the body! When that does occur, we've given it a name. We could have called it anything. We could have called it flern or applesauce. But we called it cancer. For our purposes here, cancer represents the end result of neglecting to take the proper actions to optimize the activities of the lymph system by keeping it as clean as possible. This will prevent any cells in your body from being driven crazy, and will prevent as well all the years of pain, ill health, and disease that precede that phenomenon.

But it's instructive to look at one example in depth, and I've decided to use breast cancer as that example. The first reason is that breast cancer is always associated in one's mind with the lymph nodes, and the lymph system is our main subject.

The second reason is this: Ask the next ten women whose paths you cross what their greatest health fear is. Don't be surprised if all ten, without hesitation, say breast cancer, which for most women is the health issue of the age; so much so that it is being referred to as "the other epidemic." If you were to add together all deaths from breast cancer, all deaths from all other forms of cancer, all deaths from AIDS, diabetes, and in fact, all causes of death of women by disease, they would not even come close to equaling the number of deaths from cardiovascular disease alone. But it is breast cancer that women dread the most. Why? That's not hard to figure out. All you have to do is compare the treatment and aftermath of treatment associated with heart disease to that of cancer. It's like the difference between being bitten by a mosquito and being mauled by a grizzly bear.

THE SPECTER OF BREAST CANCER

If your doctor reports that your cholesterol level is much too high and there is far too much fatty plaque in your arteries, that's not good news, because it puts you at high risk of having a heart attack. Hearing such a diagnosis would certainly alarm you, but the fear you might experience from such a diagnosis is like a stroll on the beach compared to what the words "you have cancer" evoke. After all, the treatment to ward off the heart attack is pretty straightforward. Stop pumping so much fat and cholesterol through your arteries; cut down on your salt, fried foods, tobacco, and alcohol consumption; and include a moderate amount of regular aerobic exercise in your routine. That's basically it. Not so with cancer.

The treatment for cancer can be as agonizing as the disease itself. Between the painful, disfiguring surgery; the radiation that can burn holes in your skin; and the chemotherapy, which is the most excruciatingly painful treatment ever devised for any disease, the overall impact of being told you have cancer is tantamount to being told you have to pay a visit to hell and duel the devil with burning pitchforks. That's for cancer in general. A diagnosis of breast cancer for a woman is worse yet because it has all the negatives associated with cancer and its treatment plus the ordeal of having one or both breasts removed. For some women, this can be the most devastating part of having breast cancer.

We're not talking about the removal of some nondescript organ here. Remove a gall bladder, a spleen, an appendix, and yes, these operations are painful, and having surgery, any surgery, is unnerving. But with rest and recuperation, the scars from these operations heal and life goes on pretty much as it did before. Remove a woman's breast and there's another whole set of variables that come into play. The psychological and emotional scars can last long after the physical ones have healed. The removal of a breast goes to the very heart of a woman's self-image.

Let's face it: Certainly in America and a good portion of the rest of the world, there is a fixation on women's breasts. Anyone not aware of that must be visiting from another planet.

The female form, of which the breasts are a most significant feature, has been celebrated in art, music, and poetry throughout history. A woman's breasts are deeply and profoundly associated with her femininity, her sexuality, her body image, her feeling of self-esteem and beauty. Women have told me that they felt afraid that their husbands might not think they were pretty after the loss of their breasts. They no longer feel whole and attractive. This is enormously disconcerting to a women in a way I am certain no man could possibly comprehend.

WHY BREAST CANCER?

In 1979 I had what was for me a life-changing encounter with breast cancer. Because of that experience, I knew that I would someday write something about the subject. I had been studying the field of Natural Hygiene for nine years and the publication of *Fit for Life* was still six years off. I was as convinced then as I am today that people who understood and practiced the principles of Natural Hygiene, even moderately, could ensure for themselves a long, pain-free, disease-free life.

Since 1971 I had seen, firsthand, hundreds of people do the same by following the simple principles of Natural Hygiene I outlined for them in one-on-one counseling sessions. I loved talking about health to anyone who would listen and my enthusiasm for the subject was boundless. I welcomed any challenge from people to show them how they could heal even the most seemingly catastrophic problems. I had seen so many examples of individuals overcoming serious health problems that my excitement for the subject was often catalyst enough for people to start making the simple changes I suggested. I had, and still have, the utmost confidence that because the human body is self-repairing and self-healing, it can, given the right environment for healing, overcome any ailment so long as it has not suffered irreparable damage.

This was precisely my frame of mind when I received a phone call that day in 1979 from a woman to whom I had spoken on several occasions about the beautiful and remarkable healing capabilities of the human body. Our conversations must have made an impression on her because she was calling me from the hospital. It was obvious from her voice that she was highly agitated. Her voice was so shaky and she was so upset I could hardly understand her. A mammogram had detected a rather large lump in her breast, about the size of a walnut.

Part of the problem was that her physician was there at the phone with her berating her for being so foolish as to call "some nutritional friend" for advice when he had just finished telling her that she must make arrangements at that moment for the removal of her breast or she would die!

Now, try to picture this. She goes to her doctor to find out what, if anything, was found on her mammogram and he shows her a huge lump and then proceeds to scare the juices out of her by telling her that without an immediate mastectomy she would die.

He did no biopsy, no tests, no anything. He didn't know if cancer was present or not. He didn't say that she *might* die or that with a lump that size the chances were that she had cancer and she *could* die. No. He said, no mastectomy and you're dead!

So she tells him she knows someone who knows a lot about nutrition and she wants to call him first and he erupts at her. "How could you do something so stupid when your life is at stake? This is no time for nutrition, this is time for surgery. You had better do what I say and stop messing around." He was standing next to her at the phone harassing her while she was trying to tell me what was going on. It was a real scene, believe me. Finally, I said to her that if she had a lump in her breast as big as she described, it had been growing for some ten to fifteen years at least. No matter what she decided to do, she certainly could take twenty-four to forty-eight hours to go home, reflect, talk to friends, and make a rational decision without her doctor yelling in her face that either she listens to him or dies! I suggested that she hang up the phone, tell her doctor that she would call him in a day or two, and come directly to my office so that I could tell her about an option she will never hear from her doctor.

Within an hour, she was in my office. She looked horrible. Her face was ashen and there was terror in her eyes that was so obvious you could have sliced it up and served it on a platter. Her voice was still shaky, and as soon as she started to talk, she began to cry uncontrollably. I assumed she was crying because she had found out she might have cancer, and might have to undergo surgery or chemotherapy, or both, and she was scared. In fact, it wasn't so much the cancer and treatment that upset her; it was her fear of being cut with a knife. Now, I'm not just talking about the normal fear or apprehension one might have about being operated on. No, she had such a paralyzing fear of being cut that for her, *anything* would be preferable to submitting to surgery.

I told her that Natural Hygiene, my field of study, had an entirely different perspective on lumps in the breast from traditional medicine. I explained the lymph system to her (which is invariably involved with lumps in the breast), and suggested that she take the Natural Hygiene approach to getting rid of the lump. In four or five weeks, I said, she would have absolute evidence as to whether or not the approach was successful. At that time, she would definitely see whether her lump was the same size, or whether it was larger or smaller. Since she would have preferred to do nothing rather than undergo surgery, she was willing to try anything that did not involve being cut.

The first thing I did was to fill her with a positive feeling about her body and its ability to heal itself. Her doctor's message that she was going to die was not exactly the best jumping-off place for self-healing. I explained to her that success depended upon certain dietetic maneuvering that would allow her lymph system to repair and heal itself. She promised me that she was extremely disciplined and would follow my advice without the slightest variation.

When she left my office, she was smiling and filled with hope. I advised her practically every day and she followed my suggestions implicitly. Within the first ten days she was certain that the lump had decreased somewhat in size and it was no longer tender to the touch. In three or four weeks her lump went from the size of a walnut to the size of a dime. In another four weeks, it was gone. *Gone!* She had another mammogram and there was not a trace to be found.

Of course my friend was overjoyed. You couldn't make her stop smiling with a gun. As far as she was concerned, she had been given her life back. One of the very first things she did was to call her doctor with the good news and to get a copy of the original mammogram so I could have the two, one showing the lump, the other showing nothing.

Now, most people would assume that upon learning about his patient's nonsurgical removal of a large breast lump, her doctor would walk barefoot over hot coals and broken glass to find out how she had accomplished this feat so he could share the information with his patients and colleagues. You would think he would want to trumpet the good news from the highest mountain. Well, in fact, my friend's doctor would not even take a phone call from her! He was angry at her for ignoring his advice! His secretary told her that it would be best if she were to find another physician. And no, she could not have a copy of the original mammogram.

I lost contact with my friend and did not see her again until several years later. She was still smiling, and she looked great. In the two months I had worked with her, she had lost about 30 pounds and she had obviously kept it off. More important, there were no more lumps in her breasts. In terms of my goal to educate people about how to ensure their own good health, she told me the greatest thing I could have ever hoped to hear. She said that she no longer felt as if her own body was a stranger to her or that the workings of her body were out of her realm of understanding. She felt in charge and in control of her health. When-ever she put on weight she didn't want or started to feel unwell, she knew exactly what to do to turn the situation around. She thanked me profusely for what I had done for her, not realizing that what her words had done for me was equally great.

Another friend of mine had had breast cancer before we met, and the treatment utterly ruined her life. She had a tiny lump in her right breast checked out and it did have cancer cells in it. She wanted to remove only the lump (lumpectomy) and leave the breast intact. But her doctor told her she would die if she didn't have the breast removed. After she agreed, her physician recommended that while she was having her right breast removed, she should just go ahead and have her left breast removed too. The reasoning was, if cancer appears in one breast, there is a certain likelihood that it could appear in the other breast as well. "Why take a chance of going through this again? Let's just get rid of both of them in one fell swoop and then you'll never have to worry about breast cancer again. And, oh yes, while we're at it, we'll remove all your lymph nodes from your chest and both your arms as a *precautionary* measure."

She listened and had a total of *seven* surgeries, including a radical mastectomy on one of her breasts. She lost everything she owned because she had no insurance and had to pay for everything out of her pocket. Her body was a mass of ugly scars and she was bankrupt. All because of a tiny lump in one of her breasts the size of a garden pea!

Now, you may be thinking something like, "Hey, cancer is cancer. No matter what size it was, it had to be dealt with." Dealt with, yes. But in a far saner and more sensible way. Not the all-out assault that is overkill in the extreme and which, unfortunately, has become standard medical treatment. By the end of this book you will see that the appearance of a lump in your breast, whether the size of a pea or a walnut, may be no reason to have your body mutilated and disfigured and then bombarded with the deadliest and most harmful treatments known: radiation and chemotherapy. This is especially so considering that members of the medical profession, the experts in the field, admit that they don't even know what breast cancer is. They don't know what causes it, they don't know how to cure it, and they don't know how to prevent it. So, to compensate for this total lack of knowledge, the cancer is attacked with a vengeance, in the hope that an assault on the body will somehow exorcise the cancer without killing the patient. This overly aggressive treatment is like demolishing an entire city because there is a criminal hiding in it somewhere.

These two experiences made me wonder how many other women were being bulldozed into unnecessary surgery with fear. How many women were having their lives torn apart because their doctors were aware of only one course of action: surgery followed by chemotherapy and radiation. I started to collect everything I could on breast cancer for the next fifteen years, and the results of what I learned are presented to you here.

It would probably be the greatest understatement ever uttered to say that women, all women, would do practically anything to avoid ever having to deal with breast cancer, its treatment, and its aftermath. There is one way and one way only to ensure that: prevention! It goes without saying that if women knew how to prevent breast cancer, they would do whatever they had to do. But so far, that information has not been forthcoming. The subject has been made complicated, no doubt about that, so women rely on the advice of those people who have been designated as "experts" in the field. But you are only getting part of the story. There is another whole side of it that has yet to come to light. All you're being told about is the deadliness of cancer, its pervasiveness, and the dreadful statistics that are daily being racked up. The fear! People weren't put on earth to have to live in fear of their own bodies! That is a totally unnatural and unnecessary situation that can be changed. Perhaps you know the old saying, "If there is no change, then there is no change." Vibrant health *is* possible to attain, and change is a key factor in bringing it about.

DISRUPTING THE STATUS QUO: GOOD FOR YOUR HEALTH

Change is a most interesting phenomenon. On the one hand, we all want change. We need it, we cherish it, we demand it. Imagine a world without changes such as electricity, airplanes, telephones, computers, televisions, and automobiles. Moreover, without regular and significant change, life would become unbearably boring. On the other hand, the new information that heralds theses changes we crave is, all too frequently, met with negativity and resistance. Nowhere is this more prevalent than in the sciences, the place where you would least expect it. History is rife with examples to prove this strange irony:

- From Galileo being vilified for pointing out that the sun, not the earth, is the center of the universe, to Dr. Ignaz Semmelweis being hounded out of his profession for suggesting that doctors wash their hands before surgery.
- From a time when the medical experts of the day warned that washing the entire body more than once a week was harmful, to suggesting that patients spend time in stables where they could inhale the fumes from animal dung to help heal tuberculosis.
- From refusing water to fever patients because it would be hurtful, to suggesting that fresh air would be injurious to the bedridden.

- From the admonition to eat only well-cooked food, as fresh food would be detrimental, to suggesting that bananas, being such a potent drug, should be available only by prescription.
- And the granddaddy of them all, the idea that blood should be drained from the sick to make them well.

All the above "established, proven methods" were eventually thrown on the junk heap of history, but not before the new information that brought about their change was obstinately, sometimes violently, resisted. Consider the fact that over *98 percent* of everything that has ever been learned has been replaced with new information, and you can see that resisting new information is both foolish and futile.

Much of today's barbaric treatment of women who develop lumps in their breasts needs to be thrown on that same junk heap. And you can be certain that there will be resistance to this change as well. But it doesn't matter, because this is a change that is inevitable. When you consider that the only change in breast cancer over the last hundred years is that the problem has become progressively worse, it becomes clear that this situation is screaming out for change. The only surefire way to rescue women from what is coming to be known as "the other epidemic" is to stop focusing on early detection and treatment and start focusing on prevention.

There are millions of women living in fear, biding their time waiting for the axe to fall. They're afraid of their bodies, afraid that their bodies will turn against them. Afraid of cancer. Afraid to get a mammogram for fear of what it may reveal. I know women who for a week or more before they're scheduled for a mammogram are nervous wrecks. By the time they have the mammogram and are waiting for the results, it's everything they can do not to keel over from fright. If the result is negative, the sigh of relief is as though they have just had a death sentence commuted. But that fear sits in the back of their minds, building until the next mammogram or, God forbid, a lump appears in one of their breasts. That is no way to live. It is something that must change. It can change, and if I have anything to do with it, it *will* change.

Women are being made to unnecessarily worry, anguish, live in fear, and suffer immeasurable pain. It simply does not have to be the case. The only reason it is, is because the true nature of lumps in the breast is not understood. The measures women can take to prevent them, or quickly remove them if they develop, are unknown to them. Women have been whipped into such a frenzy of fear that the mere mention of the diagnosis "breast cancer" fills them with horror and dread, and invariably results in them prematurely and unnecessarily "going under the knife." This fear is so intense that women are increasingly having both of their breasts removed before there is any sign whatsoever of cancer or *before* there is even a lump![50]

Women have choices outside of surgery, chemotherapy, and radiation and they are not being told about them. This book is going to change all that. If a woman learns about her options and still chooses to go the traditional medical route, so be it. At least she had the chance to consider other options. But to not even be given the opportunity to *hear* about her choices, while being pressured, bulldozed, and terrorized into surgery, as though it was the only viable course of action, is outrageous and entirely unacceptable. It would be one thing if the incidence of, and death rate from, breast cancer were steadily decreasing, but the exact opposite is true. It has been getting worse and worse for more than *fifty years!* In light of both this and the fact that those in charge don't know what causes breast cancer, let alone what to do about it, I would think that another course of action, other than the one that has failed so miserably to date, would be welcomed with open arms—*and minds!*

There are simple, concrete actions women can take to *dramatically* reduce their chances of ever developing breast cancer and, equally important, steps they can take to remove lumps from the breast without ever undergoing surgery—steps that prove themselves relatively quickly, so that any and all other forms of treatment would still be available to them if need be. But you should know that your first line of defense can eliminate the problem before it becomes a problem, with no surgery, radiation, or chemotherapy. You have been blessed from birth with common sense, logic, and basic instincts to help you and to guide you. You're far more capable of discerning what is best for you than you have been led to believe.

I am telling you that breast cancer does not have to be the killer that it is; that the number of women dying from the disease can be dramatically decreased; that the majority of surgical procedures, including mastectomies, can be eliminated; that the number of diagnoses of breast cancer can be drastically reduced; that there are steps you can take to protect yourself and prevent lumps from developing or from turning cancerous if they do; that you can live your life free of the fear that you may become a breast cancer casualty.

Now, there are those who will likely take issue with my contention that breast cancer (or prostate cancer, or colon cancer, etc.) is a lot less complicated and a lot easier to prevent than we've been led to believe. Issues will be raised about my credentials. Who am I to say these things? Where did I study? What proof do I have?

That I'm not a medical doctor is in my favor. And yours. It afforded me the opportunity to study before-the-fact treatment instead of after-the-fact treatment. But because I didn't study in a formal, traditional setting does not mean I didn't study. I followed the advice of Mark Twain, who said, "Never allow schooling to interfere with your education." I didn't. I never felt a need to legitimize myself with a piece of paper. I only wanted to learn everything I could, any way I could, and then let the results of my work legitimize me. In my opinion, the significance of formal, traditional "book learnin'" is equaled in importance by experience and observation, of which I have thirty years' worth.

Actually, what I have studied or not studied is irrelevant. The only thing of relevance and importance is whether the information in this book can help you prevent disease and experience vibrant health; the only thing that matters is, does it work? That's why I am telling you not only about my own experience, but of the experience and observations of doctors who use these principles in their practices with thousands of patients.

At the end of the day, however, either it will prove itself to you or it won't. All the experts in the world could praise a program or treatment up one side and down the other and it may not work. Or they could ridicule a program or treatment and it could be just the answer for some individuals. It happens all the time. If you can, with absolutely no risk to yourself, try something that may prove to be a godsend, and there is no downside, why would you *not* try it?

PREVENTION VERSUS EARLY DETECTION

I wrote this book to empower you, to free you, to put you in charge so that you can live your life with the confidence of knowing that you are not going to become a medical statistic. Worry and fear can be cast aside and become a thing of the past. And I am not telling you this just for effect or to give you false hope. *You can prevent disease!!*

I want you to be very clear on something. Just because the people you have been turning to for answers don't have any does not mean that there are no answers, or that because they don't have any, no one does. There *are* answers and there are plenty of people all over the world who have discovered this for themselves. It is not a closed club; you can join their ranks. The only thing preventing you from learning how to live a life free of disease, or from the fear of developing disease, is a lack of information. My sincerest wish is for this book to change that for you.

You are being told from every quarter that early detection is the key factor in combating breast cancer. Hogwash! *Prevention* is the key factor in combating breast cancer, or any cancer. Early detection is defeatist and negative. Buying into the idea that early detection is the most important aspect of combating cancer is admitting and accepting that there is nothing you can do except wait until *after* you have the disease. Then your fate lies in the hope that you will require the very least amount of disfiguring surgery, and the least amount of brutalizing chemotherapy and/or radiation. Prevent the problem from occurring in the first place and there is nothing to detect. That is why this book is first and foremost a book about prevention. Respect and admiration for your body has to replace your fear of it. A brand-new awareness of how magnificently capable your body is in ensuring its own well-being is essential.

"THE OTHER EPIDEMIC"

One of the most important steps in overcoming a problem, any problem, is to know that there *is* a problem. In that regard, I think a brief overview of the present status of breast cancer research and treatment is in order. Since women are looking to the experts for answers and direction, it may come as a cold, hard shot of reality to learn that the experts themselves are in just as much of a quandary over breast cancer as you. They're stumped! They want to get a handle on the disease, of course, and they *are* trying, but they are virtually incapable of supplying you with the answers you so desperately need and want. Of course, the experts will never openly admit this because such an admission would cause widespread panic. But facts are facts and the truth of what I am saying is absolute and easily proven, as you shall shortly see.

One of the most disturbing facts is that for the last fifty years at least, the problem of breast cancer has done nothing but get worse. Not only here in the United States but throughout countries rich and poor, industrial and rural, the incidence of breast cancer is on the rise. Breast cancer is the most common form of cancer in women. Approximately 185,000 women are diagnosed with breast cancer in the United States every year. Of those, approximately 46,000 die.[51] (By the way, the numbers for prostate cancer are almost the same.) Every twelve minutes, day and night, another woman dies. Overall, cancer claims the life of another person *every minute.*

Since 1950, the incidence of breast cancer has increased 60 percent, making it one of the fastest-growing killer diseases in the nation.[52] Since 1960, the number of American women who died from breast cancer is more than twice the number of all Americans killed in World War I, World War II, the Korean War, the Vietnam War, and the Gulf War. Half of these women died in the ten years from 1983 to 1993,[53] which shows the death rate *increasing* as time goes by. In 1962, one in twenty women got breast cancer. In 1982, the number was one in eleven.[54] In 1993, the number was one in eight,[55] and in the year 2000 it was one in seven women but returned to one in eight as of 2020.[56]

On ABC's "Nightline," Cindy Pearson, program director for the National Women's Health Network, was asked, "Is there a breast cancer epidemic in this country?" Her reply: "What else would you call a condition that has increased in incidence every year for the last forty years with no explanation and no effective cure? I think there's nothing else to call it but an epidemic."[57]

DOCUMENTING CANCER

You will notice that a lot of my supporting documentation comes from common, everyday sources. Not that I don't also use scientific journals. I do. But frankly, the vast majority do not read these journals because they are written in obscure, scientific jargon. I prefer to use the sources that you are most familiar with: television, radio, newspapers, and magazines. Also, when it comes to scientific studies that are published in scholarly journals, it is well known that any premise whatsoever can be "scientifically proven." Depending on who is funding the studies and what outcome is desired even two opposite views can be "proven."

A classic example of science *proving* both sides of an issue is found in the *New England Journal of Medicine,*[58] easily one of the most prestigious and well respected of all medical journals. In one issue, there are two articles on the subject of heart attacks in women. One article "proves" that giving female hormones to postmenopausal women can substantially protect them against heart attacks. The second article, equally well substantiated, "proves" that giving hormones to postmenopausal women can substantially increase their chances of having a heart attack. Now mind you, these two contradictory studies weren't in the same journal on different dates, two years apart. They were in the very same issue!

How often do you sit down and read scientific or scholarly journals? Probably never. The average person will read newspapers or magazines several times a week and never even see a scientific journal. I consider it my role to point out what you may be missing in the articles you're reading or programs you're watching or listening to. You see, you may read an article on cancer and be lulled into thinking that more is being done or more progress is being made than is actually the case.

Frequently, I read an article in the newspaper that is filled with what may happen, or what might take place, or what is perhaps the case, or what outcome is hoped for, or what avenues of study look promising, or that researchers are encouraged by prospects that can and should be pursued further, or that the answer is just around the corner, and on and on and on. Buried deep underneath all the wished-for progress are perhaps one or two sentences that reveal the true state of affairs in terms of actual progress being made. The thing is, most people never notice these few sentences. They are not highlighted or embellished, and so get lost amid the fluff. People just don't have the trained eye to seek out and find these buried jewels that give a more honest and accurate evaluation of the overall situation. When these sentences are scrutinized more closely, an unmistakable pattern emerges. I have been playing this hide-and-seek game for thirty years. Those few sentences of worth jump out at me now like neon lights that are flashing away in rapid fire.

THE EXPERTS ARE BAFFLED

To illustrate just how baffled the experts are about cancer, I have extracted some of these statements and present them below. These are revealing statements made by people who are in the best possible position to know the real status of progress being made in the battle against breast cancer. (Although the following examples refer to breast cancer, I could just as easily be using any other type of cancer to illustrate my point. Remember, cancer, *all* cancer, is woefully misunderstood. Any one of the following quotations could easily be about prostate cancer, for example.)

There are two things we don't know about breast cancer.
We don't know the cause and we don't know the cure.[59]

> —Nancy Brinker, Chairwoman,
> President's Special Commission
> on Breast Cancer

Nobody knows what causes breast cancer, nobody
knows how to prevent it, and nobody knows how to
cure it.[60]

> —Linda Ellerbee,
> Narrating an ABC special on breast
> cancer

We don't know what causes it . . . there's no way to
prevent it.[61]

> —Jane Pauley,
> Narrating a PBS special on breast
> cancer

No one knows how to prevent it, and the mortality rate
from breast cancer has not improved for decades.
Researchers say it is also disconcerting that the rates
have remained so high.[62]

> —*The New York Times*

So many questions, one answer: We don't know. Breast
cancer—never have so many been given so much conflicting advice and so few definitive solutions.[63]

> —Cokie Roberts,
> ABC "Nightline"

Throughout countries rich and poor, industrial and rural, breast cancer incidence is on the rise. No one knows what's fueling that increase.[64]

—*Science News*

This continual rise in breast cancer is unexplained. We have some hints at what's causing it, but we don't know the whole story and we also don't know how to stop it or how to cure it when it occurs.[65]

—Cindy Pearson, Program Director,
National Women's Health Network

We really don't know what causes breast cancer. We don't really even have a clue what causes breast cancer.[66]

—Dr. Susan Love,
breast surgeon, author of
Dr. Susan Love's Breast Book,
past Assistant Clinical Professor at
Harvard Medical School, Director of
U.C.L.A.'s Breast Center

Women are very frightened by breast cancer and there is nothing they can do to prevent it.[67]

—Maryann Napoli,
Associate Director, Center for
Medical Consumers in New York

If we knew how to prevent breast cancer, believe me we would have done it. We don't know how.[68]

> —John Laszlo, M.D.,
> Senior Vice-President for Research,
> American Cancer Society

We don't know the natural history of this disease. We don't know whether treatment is necessary and we don't know if it works.[69]

> —Dr. H. Gilbert Welsh,
> Senior Research Associate,
> Department of Veterans Affairs

It's horribly frustrating because I tend to like to look at prevention. If we knew what caused it, we could figure out how to prevent it, but we don't know yet.[70]

> —Dr. Janet Osuch,
> Breast cancer specialist at Michigan
> State University

Scientists do not understand much about the causes of breast cancer. So while they can detect and treat breast cancer, they do not know how to prevent it.[71]

> —Robert Bazell,
> NBC News science correspondent

In the above quotations, did you grasp the most important message? Did you notice that every "expert" categorically states that "we don't know," or "no one knows"? Be assured, they would likely prefer not to admit this, but what choice did they have, when the evidence confirming the accuracy of these statements is so overwhelming? It is extremely important that you take the above comments seriously. That is the only way you will be moved to take the actions necessary to protect yourself. I know that many people will be stunned to learn that so little is actually known about breast cancer and that many of the reports of headway made in research have only been what the researchers *think* may be the case, or what they *hoped* would be the case. After all, you have to be told something. Imagine your reaction if you asked cancer experts a pertinent question on breast cancer and all they could do was turn their palms up, scrunch up their shoulders, and say, "Sorry, but we just don't know." So instead, they tell you what they think *may* be the answer. What you're getting is conjecture and speculation, nothing concrete. Over time people tend to see what *may* be as what *is,* and they are lulled into complacency.

Let's look at the three most important issues in question.

1. *They don't know the cause.* Without question, there are risk factors, but what are they? You're probably familiar with the ones that are mentioned most often: the hormone estrogen, early menstruation, late menopause, pregnancy late in life, never having a pregnancy, birth control pills, heredity, and environment (which comprises a lot of factors including pesticides, other chemicals, and diet). Remember, these are guesses. None have been absolutely proven to cause cancer. They may all play a role or none may play a role. They may only be contributing factors . . . or not. On a nationally broadcast program on breast cancer, Jane Pauley states that, "Most women who get breast cancer do not fit into any high-risk category. There's no way to predict who will get it."[72] Breast surgeon and author Dr. Susan Love states that, "Eighty percent of the women who are diagnosed with breast cancer have no risk factors whatsoever, except being a woman."[73] Based on that, one could say that the only absolute risk factor is being a woman.

It's interesting that most women seem to think that the biggest risk factor is having a family member who has had breast cancer. Equally interesting is the fact that only 5 percent of breast cancer cases can be linked to a family history of the disease.[74] That figure is probably more a reflection of coincidence or the law of averages than a major risk factor.

Also, a recent study found that when a woman moves to a new country, her risk of dying of breast cancer will rise or fall to match the death rate of women in the newly adopted country. This suggests that environmental factors, such as diet, have more impact than family history. The study contradicts current notions that most of a woman's risk of breast cancer is set by the time she reaches puberty or early adulthood. Dr. Noel S. Weiss, professor of epidemiology at the University of Washington School of Public Health in Seattle, says, "The importance of this study is that it reinforces our notion that your risk of breast cancer isn't something you're born with."[75]

2. *They don't know the cure.* Although the bulk of research dollars are spent on the search for a cure, there is no magic bullet for breast cancer, or any cancer, that, once administered, makes the disease disappear, or we would surely know about it. Yet we hear about the "cure rate" of breast cancer patients. If a woman is still alive five years after her cancer is first treated, she falls into the category of "the cured." To put it mildly, this is a great big stretch of the word. Surviving five years is hardly a cure. Especially when you consider that twenty years after diagnosis, breast cancer is the cause of death for 88 percent of those women who have died.[76] In other words, 88 out of 100 died of the disease they were "cured" of.

The five-year survival statistic is completely arbitrary. It is a "line drawn in the sand," its only meaning being that the patient has managed to survive five years after diagnosis. It hardly means cure. Every time I hear the five-year survival mentioned, I'm reminded of a movie I once saw, in which tribal warriors capture their enemies and make them run a gauntlet of men who beat them with punches, kicks, and clubs. The prisoners are told if they can make it to the end of the gauntlet, they can live. Some did make it, although they were crippled for life. But I guess it was better than being killed. Women who are diagnosed with breast cancer not only have to deal with the progression of the disease itself, but they also have to withstand the treatment, which, as we know, can be horrific. If they submit to surgery, radiation, and chemotherapy, referred to by Andrea Martin, executive director of the Breast Cancer Fund, as "the slash, burn and poison routine of cancer treatment," it will take its toll. At the end of the five years, a woman could be disfigured, bald, psychologically crushed, emotionally bankrupt, in constant pain, and on drugs to quell the pain and be declared "cured." I don't think so.

3. *They don't know how to prevent it.* Of the three, this is the issue that is most self-evident. If there were any means in place by which to prevent breast cancer, the problem would not be getting worse every passing year. The irony is that prevention, which without question is the most important aspect of breast cancer, is given scant, if any, attention whatsoever. Yes, scads of lip service is given to the subject of prevention, but that's it. The vast majority of money spent on breast cancer research, which is many billions of dollars annually, is spent on after-the-fact research, such as early detection and treatment.

The National Cancer Institute in Bethesda, Maryland, receives approximately $1.8 billion a year in federal money for research, and a paltry 5 percent is spent on prevention. And only 5 percent of *that* ($\frac{1}{4}$ of 1 percent of the total) is spent on breast cancer prevention.[77] That's not just peanuts, that's barely peanut skins! Why is spending on breast cancer research so low? Why, when no one, and I mean no one, could possibly dispute the fact that prevention is the key to ending, or at least to diminishing, the pain and suffering of breast cancer, is so little attention actually paid to it? It is a troubling question, and the answer, at least in part, is not very pleasant to think about. I know it's going to sound cynical and coldhearted, but a big part of the reason has to do with money. There's simply more money to be had in chasing cures and selling drugs than in teaching lifestyle changes to prevent disease. Ouch!

I know how much it must disturb you to hear that, but to deny that money is a factor is foolish. I'm not suggesting or even remotely hinting that there are people sitting around saying things like, "The heck with prevention, there's no money in it. Let's concentrate on what will make the most bucks." No way. But when we talk about the money generated by the health-care industry in the United States, we're talking about the biggest moneymaking machine there is.

Most people think that the United States spends more money on national defense than on anything else. The U.S. does spend a lot: about $300 billion a year. But multiply that by 3 and you still don't equal what is spent on health care, which remember, clocks in at a mind-boggling $1 trillion a year. That's 1 thousand billion! This is going to sound heartless as hell, but who stands to lose the most money if cancer is prevented? The cancer establishment! Consider the words of Dr. Samuel Epstein, professor of occupational and environmental medicine at the School of Public Health, University of Chicago Medical Center: "The cancer establishment, the National Cancer Institute, the American Cancer Society, and the pharmaceutical companies associated with them are virtually indifferent or hostile to problems of cancer prevention."[78] Can you think of any legitimate reason why a pharmaceutical company, or anyone for that matter, should be "hostile" toward cancer prevention? I can't either.

THE EARLY DETECTION TRAP

So, having acknowledged, admitted, and accepted that the cause, cure, and prevention of breast cancer have eluded them, the experts find themselves in the unenviable position of having to offer up *something.* They can ill afford to look perplexed and give us the old "Gee, I don't know what to tell ya." And what they have pinned all their hopes on, and yours, is what is referred to as "early detection." With nowhere else to turn, all energy is being directed toward early detection.

As part of President Bill Clinton's attempt to provide universal health care, the government asked experts to devise a strategy to deal with the growing incidence of and death from breast cancer. In an address at the opening session of a conference on breast cancer at the National Institutes of Health, in Washington, D.C., Donna E. Shalala, Health and Human Services Secretary, stated that, "The plan must address why the incidence of breast cancer is steadily rising, and what action we must take to detect breast cancer earlier."[79] Discussing breast cancer and women's options, Dr. Timothy Johnson, ABC News medical director, says that "the only thing they [women] can do right now is to try to detect it early through self-exam, physician exam and mammography."[80] (Note the word "only.") Dr. Susan Love was asked by a woman what she could do to lower her risk of breast cancer. Dr. Love's answer was: "The only hope we have right now in terms of dealing with breast cancer is in early detection and that means mammography."[81]

The *only* hope? Not only is early detection not your only hope, it's barely any hope at all. Relying on early detection as your "only hope" is to give up and admit defeat. *Early detection means you have cancer!* Don't accept that.

You know, I read lots of material from many support groups that work with breast cancer patients and also try to bring awareness of the seriousness of breast cancer to both the public and agencies that allocate money for breast cancer research. A theme that seems to run through virtually all this material is a call to arms for women. They want women to speak up and speak out, to fight back, to get angry and *demand* something be done. Good idea! And if you want something to really get angry about, get angry about being told that your "only hope" in dealing with breast cancer is to sit around and wait until you get it, then hope you detect it before it kills you. Because that is precisely what you are being told to do. After all is said and done, after all the talk and posturing about what's been done and what's being done, after all the billions spent and research conducted, all the most highly advanced and technologically superior medical machine in the world can tell you is, in effect . . . nothing! Your last glimmer of hope, your last resort and refuge, lies in a test with the efficiency and accuracy of a coin toss: mammography.

MAMMOGRAPHY: YOUR ONLY HOPE?

All attention and focus as relates to the subject of breast cancer is directed toward mammography. Why? Because there's nothing else to offer. Creating a hubbub around mammography gives the appearance that something is being done about breast cancer. And so now there is what is described in the *New York Times* as "One of the most contentious disputes in medicine."[82] Another article in the *Times* describes the controversy surrounding mammography guidelines as a "wrenching" and "impassioned" debate among the experts.[83] And what is this debate that has captured the headlines? It focuses on this question: Should women under the age of fifty have regular mammograms?

According to a number of studies, if women over age fifty have mammograms every one to two years, their risk of dying of breast cancer is reduced by one-third.[84] But there are no such studies to prove that the same is true for women in their forties. This controversy has flared on and off since the seventies.[85] The United States stands virtually alone in recommending mammography for women in their forties.[86] "The eight-nation Euro-pean Group for Breast Cancer opposes it on the basis that there is no demonstrated benefit."[87] The "experts" in the United States seem to be equally divided, with opponents saying there is no scientific evidence to support mammography for women in their forties. And since the tissue in a younger woman's breast is far denser than the tissue in the breasts of a woman in her fifties or older, the possibility of high rates of false positives, which can lead to unnecessary treatments, is greatly increased.

Dr. Suzanne W. Fletcher, coeditor of the *Annals of Internal Medicine,* and her husband, Dr. Robert H. Fletcher, write, "Medical scientists and physicians do not do modern women a service by promulgating a screening practice that medical science has not been able to substantiate after so many tries.[88] Proponents of the test for women in their forties acknowledge that there are no good scientific studies to prove the value of mammography for these women, but their argument is that there are no studies proving that they *don't* help either.

And so the dispute rages on. It's interesting that in all other matters of health care, medical experts, across the board, adamantly insist that good, hard data from scientifically sound studies be in place before tests are done. Why the exception here? If you think about it, traditional medicine has always played kind of fast and loose with women's health issues, and this appears to be another example of it. There's another factor to consider that no one *wants* to believe is influencing the decision to push for mammography for women under age fifty, but it's pretty hard to ignore. Money!

In keeping with my earlier suggestion that the money incentive is something that should always be looked at when talking about a trillion-dollar industry, I came across an interesting comment from Dr. Howard Ozer, chief of medical oncology at the University of North Carolina School of Medicine. He was being interviewed about the debate over the screening guidelines for women in their forties, and among several points he was making, he said that "the mammography business has become highly lucrative and younger women are the best customers."[89] No need to embellish on that, he makes the point better than I.

The worst part about all this is that it's a smoke screen that clouds the more important issues. Keeping the ongoing controversy of mammography for early detection in the public eye keeps women thinking about the issue, instead of the bigger, more important issue of prevention! Never allow the fact to drift from your mind that the use of mammography for early detection concerns itself with only one thing: finding a cancerous tumor in your breast. Let's not lose sight of your goal here, which isn't to locate a tumor in your breast, but to avoid ever developing one.

Actually, it would be one thing if mammography performed the service it is intended to, dependably and precisely, but there is an unsettling irony in all of this. On the one hand, you are being told, in the clearest possible language, that there is no way to prevent or cure breast cancer, so all of your faith and trust should be focused on mammography for early detection, which is being held up as your final bastion of hope. On the other hand, mammography's track record of reliability isn't exactly something that will fill you with confidence. Mammography fails to detect as much as 20 percent of all breast cancers and as much as 40 percent in women under the age of fifty,[90] and that is in the best of circumstances when all procedures involved in the test are performed with high efficiency.

Examples of how treatment was either withheld when it should have been given, or given when it should have been withheld, could fill this book. Here are a few:

- The television show "Primetime Live" tells the story of a woman who was experiencing soreness in her breast, so she had a mammogram and was told, "Everything is normal." But within eight months, the cancer that was missed grew and spread. The woman's breast had to be removed.[91]
- Another television show—"Good Morning America"— tells the tragic story of a woman who was informed that she had cancer; this diagnosis was based on a laboratory examination of tissue from her breast by a pathologist who had thirty years' experience. The woman had both

breasts removed only to find out later that she didn't have cancer.[92]

- In April 1994, a Florida woman whose left breast was removed after a misdiagnosis of cancer was awarded $2.7 million. The jury ruled that all *four* of the doctors who were involved in her diagnosis were negligent. Astonishingly, the mistake was discovered two weeks before her mastectomy, but no one spoke up.[93]

The problem with placing so much reliance on mammography for early detection lies in the fact that there are several variables that come into play at once and influence the ultimate diagnosis. If any one of these variables is inaccurate or performed incorrectly, the probability of a misdiagnosis goes way up. There are three factors that are of extreme importance: the machine taking the X-ray picture or mammogram, the technician operating the machine, and the interpretation of the film.

In 1992, ABC's "Primetime Live" conducted a four-month investigation that canvassed the country interviewing surgeons, radiologists, cancer patients, and cancer experts. What they discovered is that "there is a crisis in the quality of mammography in this country.[94] Unlike Western Europe, where there are federal regulations, the mammography business in the United States has proliferated with virtually no rules. Until very recently, there were no national quality standards. Many of the machines simply do not take good pictures and they are being used every day. In Michigan, it was discovered that 35 to 50 percent of the facilities doing mammographies were doing unacceptable work. Michigan cracked down on these faulty facilities and now has the toughest laws in the country. But only nine states have tough laws governing mammography. That means forty-one states do not!

The operators (technologists) of mammogram machines should have what can amount to two years of study in X-ray technology; this is according to Dr. Ed Hendrick, professor at the University of Colorado and top physicist at the American

College of Radiology. A crucial and complicated part of the mammography procedure is the careful placement of the breast. Since each patient is different, a technologist has to know how to compress the breast, not to mention test the machine and check the processing of the film. In one instance, "Primetime's" hidden cameras showed a nurse with only two days' training in mammography doubling as a technologist. In another office, the receptionist did mammographies and she, too, had only two days' training. In twenty-one states, technologists don't even have to be licensed. Diane Sawyer, the co-anchor of "Prime-time," said, "In a lot of states there's more supervision of pizza parlors than mammographies." And this, so you are told, is your "only hope" in dealing with breast cancer.

Here is a rather astonishing piece of information that too few women are aware of and that seriously weakens the premise that early detection is the key in avoiding becoming a breast cancer statistic. Remember that cancer cells grow at a very slow pace; it can take about ten years to even be detectable on a mammogram.[95] At that point, it is one centimeter, about the size of a pea. I want to be sure you see the full import of what I am saying: You can religiously get a mammogram every year and not have a cancer show up that has been growing in your breast for *ten* years.

And then there is the all-important issue of interpretation. A new study has raised serious questions about radiologists' reliability in reading mammograms and making recommendations about what to do when a suspicious lesion is found in the breast. The study, by researchers at Yale University School of Medicine and published in the *New England Journal of Medicine,* found that interpretations and advice given based on those interpretations vary greatly. Where one radiologist might recommend an immediate biopsy, another, looking at the same mammogram, might suggest a repeat X ray in three months, and still another might suggest waiting a year to do another mammogram.[96]

In November 1992, a landmark Canadian study on mammography—the largest study ever conducted in the world, involving 90,000 women—showed "no benefit for women under forty-nine" and it "fails to reduce breast cancer deaths among women between fifty and fifty-nine."[97] Consider the words of physician and best-selling author Dr. John McDougall: "Be-cause most of the years of cancer growth are hidden at microscopic levels, efforts toward early detection are unlikely to ever yield much success in saving lives."[98] And, "To be quite realistic, in most cases the only real beneficiaries from early detection are the health professionals. Early detection gets the patient going to the doctor earlier and, thereby, a longer total time period is available for more expensive doctor visits, hospitalizations and tests. And the patient lives no longer or better from all this well meaning effort."[99]

As more ingenious techniques are developed to detect smaller and smaller cancers, some investigators are voicing their concerns. They point out that studies show that many, if not most, early cancers do not grow large and dangerous and would never be noticed unless doctors with an early detection method went looking for them. Tiny cancers are so common that autopsy studies of middle-aged and older people have found that almost everyone's body contains them. No one can tell which early cancers are dangerous and which ones are not, and no one understands enough about the natural history of cancer to know what it means to find a tumor so small. This led Dr. Barry Kramer, associate director of the Early Detection and Community Oncology Program at the National Cancer Institute, to state, "We have to meticulously avoid the tendency to assume that early diagnosis in and of itself will make a difference."[100] After all the hoopla centered on early detection, this specialist is saying that early detection makes no difference!

Do you know what I think of every time I hear about people depending on early detection to save them from dying of cancer? I imagine two people mountain climbing, and one of them slips off the edge of a cliff and is stranded on a small ledge jutting over a 2,000-foot drop. The person above throws down a frayed old rope that looks as if it was left over from the Spanish-American War. The person on the ledge yells up that the rope doesn't look as though it will hold any weight and the person throwing the rope down says, "It's all we have, just grab hold and hope for the best." That's what you're being asked to do with mammography and early detection. On MSNBC's "Today in America," Dr. Daniel Kopans, Professor of Radiol-ogy at Harvard Medical School, was asked about this very thing and replied, "Mammography is not the ultimate solution to the problem of breast cancer in this country or around the world . . . but is the best of what we have today."[101] Fortunately, for the purposes of this book at least, mammography is irrelevant. We're not looking to detect, we're looking to prevent. And mammographies have absolutely nothing to do with prevention. Nothing!

Once again, the words of Dr. Susan Love: "What we really need is some kind of prevention of breast cancer, not finding it. We need to prevent it from happening."[102] By using the information in this book, you're taking a giant step toward preventing ever developing cancerous lumps anywhere in your body.

I want to state clearly and categorically that I am not suggesting that women stop getting regular mammograms. I am saying that I want mammography to become something else in your consciousness. I want you to see it, not as a tool to detect an existing cancer, but as a means by which you prove to yourself that you are successfully preventing cancer from getting a foothold.

Mammography will go from being a life raft thrown to a drowning person to a monitoring device to validate your success.

I could easily understand if you are upset by what you have read in this chapter. After all, it can be disconcerting to find out that the experts you are relying on for direction are as baffled about breast cancer as you are, to put it mildly. But I want you to be very clear about something: I did not share that revelation with you in order to alarm you, but to alert you to the fact that complacent reliance on the experts is not going to serve you well at this time.

I live in South Florida, where the danger of a hurricane coming through and wiping me out is a very real possibility. When I'm warned of a hurricane approaching, it is not done to scare me, it's done to give me the opportunity to take the measures necessary to save my life. It's true, I may have given you information that is upsetting, but more important, I am also going to give you the information that you need to save *your* life.

Because we live in a drug-oriented culture where we have been convinced that our salvation in all matters associated with health lies in finding the appropriate drug, people have lost sight of what prevention truly means. We have been conditioned to believe that sooner or later someone will come up with a shot or pill that will prevent breast cancer from occurring. Buying into that can cost you dearly. There's no drug, no shot, no pill, no potion that will prevent the inevitable results of negative living habits from coming to pass. And even if such a miracle *should* occur, in ten, or twenty or thirty years, what about now? Place your faith and reliance in the unparalleled wisdom and intelligence that governs your body, not the pharmaceutical industry.

Michael Sporn, director of the new National Cancer Institute laboratory devoted to intervening in precancerous stages of the disease using a combination of new therapies, states that, "Over the next twenty-five years, breast cancer will disappear like the Cheshire cat."[103] I'm all for positive thinking, but breast cancer is not going to just "disappear." There is no magic bullet. But there are actions women can take *now* to protect themselves and prevent the disease.

I do not wish to imply that this book is going to wipe out cancer. There are no such guarantees from anyone. There are some people who no matter what they do, and no matter how conscientious they are, *will* get cancer and die from it. That's a cold, hard fact of life. What I am saying is that a lot of people, a lot, will be able to avoid that fate by following the recommendations in this book.

Dr. I. Craig Henderson is a breast cancer researcher who is chief of medical oncology at the University of California in San Francisco. In an interview with the *New York Times,* he stated that, "Science often made its leaps from unexpected directions, which means that the next great advance in breast cancer may not come from breast cancer research. It is important for us to follow the clues wherever they are and to realize that the answer may not be in breast cancer directed funds."[104]

Thank you, Dr. Henderson, those are my sentiments exactly. And this book is my contribution to proving you right.

SEVEN

Health in Action

The purpose of this chapter is to look at some of the health problems that will inevitably develop long before any cells are ever driven crazy. The cells of your body are astonishingly resilient and can hold out for years on end before they actually go bonkers. But remember that those years on end can be riddled with all manner of health difficulties, many of which are signals—warnings, if you will—from the body, alerting you to the fact that the lymph system, the mechanism in the body designed to keep you well, is overburdened. If those warnings are heeded and the proper steps are taken to lower the level of toxins, the discomfort will cease. If the warnings are ignored, and the level of toxemia is allowed to build, more serious problems will most certainly develop, as the disease process trudges on, slowly but surely.

I'm going to introduce to you now yet one more new way of thinking. We tend to think of ill health and disease as things that happen haphazardly, with no rhyme or reason. People living in the exact same circumstances, in the same place, eating the same food, drinking the same water, everything the same, don't necessarily develop the same health problems. One person may develop diabetes, while another develops migraines, while another develops a skin disorder, while yet another has an organ fail, and on and on. One might conclude, therefore, that it is haphazardly determined who gets sick with what. Let me assure you that there is unity in disease just as there is with every other aspect of the human body. There is *nothing* whatsoever that is haphazard about any aspect of the human body and its functions.

You have certainly heard the old adage, "A chain is only as strong as its weakest link." So it is with the human body. Every one of the 7,000,000,000 plus people living on this planet has a weakest link. Everybody who allows their lymph systems to become overburdened with toxins will get a warning from their body in the guise of pain or ill health; *where* in the body depends on each individual's particular weakest link. So it doesn't really matter where in the body this happens, it only matters that it did happen. Sound familiar? It's exactly what I have been saying about cells being driven crazy. It doesn't matter where it happens, only that it does indeed happen. I want you to apply the same principle that cancer is cancer no matter where it shows up, to disease in general.

Of course, I can't say this is so for every single malady of the body. A person could be poisoned or breathe in asbestos or develop some skin condition from an outside influence. But apart from a few exceptions, in general, whatever goes awry in the human body is the result of toxins in the system causing some kind of disruption, resulting in pain, illness, or disease.

For those of you who may be saying something like, "Hey, you can't tell me that diabetes is the same thing as eczema!"— actually, yes, I can. I know that with one we're talking about the pancreas, an internal organ, losing its ability to properly provide insulin. With the other we're talking about the skin, an external organ, becoming itchy, red, and raw. On the surface they certainly would appear to be two completely different ailments. But that is so only if you are considering the *effects,* which have different appearances, instead of the all-important *cause,* which is the same for both. And that cause is toxemia: more toxins being produced in the body than the lymph system can break down and eliminate.

Visualize, if you will, a coastal community at the foot of a mountain, with houses all along the coast, some inland and some near the base of the mountains. If offshore, deep in the ocean, an earthquake occurs, it will send a tidal surge of water crashing right into our little coastal community. The water will destroy a certain number of houses. The earthquake sends boulders from the mountain crashing down on some other houses. And fires started by snapping electrical lines destroy yet other houses. So here we have houses destroyed by water, falling rocks, and fire. Now, fire and water are as about as different as two things can be. And boulders are like neither. The houses are destroyed by three different means. But all three had the same cause! If not for the earthquake, there would be no tidal wave, no falling boulders, and no fires. If not for toxemia, there would be no diabetes, no eczema, no fever, no cancer, virtually no disease.

Disease, ill health, pain, wherever they may appear, are merely points at which the uneliminated toxins finally overwhelmed the body's ability to contain them. By explaining one disease to you, I've explained virtually all of them. Because to prevent them, or even reverse them, toxins must be removed from the lymph system. Could it be simpler? Yet experts are regularly baffled, mystified, dumbfounded by it all explaining time after time, "We don't know," "No one knows," "The cause is unknown." That's because they think there is no unity in disease, that it is haphazard, so they are trying to find the specific cause for each and every one of the hundreds upon hundreds of different possible ailments of the human body when in actual fact there is but one: toxemia.

If you are having difficulty accepting this concept of the unity of disease, you're not alone. It's like that sometimes with new ideas and new concepts. After all, it's different from what you have ever thought. You know what an apple is, right? All your life you've known that if you wanted one of those bright red, crispy sweet pieces of fruit all you had to do was ask your friendly grocer for an apple. What if, starting tomorrow, you found out they weren't actually called apples, they're called jump ropes. "Yes, I'll have a bag of those oranges and a bag of those jump ropes." It wouldn't be easy, would it? That's a little bit like what you're being asked to do here. Accept that the only difference between most diseases is that they may appear at different places in the body, but they have the exact same root cause.

What I would also like for you to know is that the strangeness of it is fleeting. It's the natural, initial response to something so new and different. But the concept will prove itself to you over time. In thirty years I have seen how people gradually become more assured of its validity as they see, time and again, examples of how cleaning the lymph system ends pain and ill health. It's what solidified its soundness for me.

As one doctor puts it, "With the accumulation of toxic elements in the lymph system the flow of lymph can become sluggish. The fluid actually becomes thick and the T-cells and macrophages of the immune system become bogged down and don't move around as well. With a regimen that cleanses the lymph system of toxins, I have seen countless patients recover from autoimmune diseases, cancer, and chronic degenerative diseases such as arthritis. I have cancer patients who are alive nineteen years later because we worked on opening up the lymph system and restoring the immune system to proper functioning."

So many people view their health as the equivalent of walking through a minefield: "If one thing doesn't get you, another will." When you understand the principles of Natural

Hygiene, all of a sudden there are a whole heck of a lot fewer mines out there.

THE LYMPH SYSTEM IN ACTION

In order to demonstrate more specifically how the lymph system works, I need to discuss some examples, but which of all the possible ailments to choose? To even list all of them would fill this book, and of course, the whole point is that there really aren't hundreds upon hundreds of different ones. But people want to read about the specific illness they are concerned about or that ails them.

Just know that no matter what specific problem I discuss or do not discuss, the remedy is the same: use the CARE principles to clean your lymph system, and it will. After all, that is the reason this book was even written. To bring to your attention the fact that there is a mechanism in your body designed specifically to keep you well and keep you alive. And if it is cared for properly it will do exactly that. So if you don't see the exact ailment you're interested in, just know that the advice I'm giving for the ones that are mentioned, is the same I would be giving to you as well. That is because cleaning out your lymph system can only have a positive effect and result in good.

Before I dive in, I want you to have fresh in your mind the wide range of symptoms of a lymph system in distress described to you in Chapter Four. Remember my asking you to read that chapter as many times as it takes for you to be familiar with the symptoms? This might be the perfect time for you to reread it.

Recall that there are symptoms that start right off in Stage 1 and continue all the way through every stage right up to the point of cells being driven crazy. These include any type of uncharacteristic fatigue or tiredness; fitful sleep; loss of appetite; skin disorders, especially itching; pain; fever; swollen or painful glands (of course!); headaches or other body aches; irregular menstrual periods in women; any type of seemingly unprovoked irritability; and any and all types of inflammation (the itises). Any or all of the above symptoms indicate that your body is trying to get your attention by alerting you to the fact that it is marshaling its forces to protect itself from the harmful effects of uneliminated toxins. It is then incumbent upon you to clean the lymph system so that the symptoms can abate.

THE IMMUNE DISORDERS

Before the appearance of AIDS on the scene, how often did you ever hear or use the term *immune system?* Probably not at all. AIDS definitely raised our awareness of the importance of the immune system; in fact, one way or another the immune system is involved in all aspects of our health. And as I've already stated, the lymph system is the heart and soul of the immune system. So what better place for me to start than with some of the immune disorders that seemed to have dominated the 1990s, and which are a concern for most of the people I come into contact with.

1. Chronic fatigue syndrome: a complex syndrome with persistent flu-like symptoms, including fever, lymph node swelling, joint and muscle pain, and frequently mood swings and other psychological symptoms.
    By the way, the word syndrome refers to any group of symptoms for which there is no known cause, which certainly explains why there are so many of them.
    Symptoms: Overwhelming fatigue, fever, painful glands, sleep disturbances, headaches, and irritability.

Cause: Unknown.

Treatment: Drugs.

2. Lupus: a chronic disorder of the connective tissue deep in the body.

    Symptoms: Deep, unrelenting pain throughout the body, fever, joint discomfort similar to rheumatoid arthritis, loss of appetite, lymph node enlargement, headaches, irritability, absent or irregular menstrual cycles in women.

    Cause: Unknown.

    Treatment: Anti-inflammatory drugs.

3. Fibromyalgia: a chronic disorder of the musculo-skeletal system. Similar to lupus (55 percent of all fibromyalgia patients also have lupus).[105]

    Symptoms: Unrelenting pain throughout the body, particularly at "tender points" at various sites, fitful sleep, inflammation (in fact, fibromyalgia is also referred to as fibrocytis, so you know there is inflammation) and so many more symptoms it reads like an encyclopedia.

    Cause: Unknown.

    Treatment: Anti-inflammatory drugs.

4. Rheumatoid arthritis: a systemic inflammatory disease that primarily attacks the joints of the hands, arms, and feet as well as surrounding muscles, tendons, ligaments, and blood vessels.

    Symptoms: Fatigue, loss of appetite, inflammation, persistent low-grade fever, disease of the lymph nodes.

    Cause: Unknown.

    Treatment: Anti-inflammatory drugs.

5. Atopic dermatitis: a chronic skin disorder characterized by inflammation and itching.

   Symptoms: Unrelenting itchiness that can develop into lesions and become scaly due to scratching.

   Cause: Unknown.

   Treatment: Drugs.

6. Scleroderma: connective tissue disorder with inflammation affecting the skin, blood vessels, skeletal muscles, and internal organs.

   Symptoms: Pain, blanched or discolored skin, possible ulceration on the tips of toes or fingers that can lead to gangrene.

   Cause: Unknown.

   Treatment: Drugs.

7. Vasculitis: a broad spectrum of disorders characterized by inflammation and/or destruction of blood vessels.

   Symptoms: Pain, inflammation, headache, oral ulcers, skin lesions.

   Cause: Unknown.

   Treatment: Anti-inflammatory drugs.

8. Reiter's syndrome: painful inflammation of the urethra or penis.

   Symptoms: Difficult, urgent, or frequent urination; blood, mucus, or pus in the urine; skin lesions such as small ulcers on the tip of the penis; fever; loss of appetite.

   Cause: Unknown.

   Treatment: Anti-inflammatory drugs.

9. Ankylosing spondylitis: a chronic inflammatory disease affecting the spine and adjacent soft tissue.

Symptoms: Pain (usually lower back); inflammation of shoulders, hips, and knees; mild fatigue; fever; loss of appetite.

Cause: Unknown.

Treatment: Anti-inflammatory drugs.

10. Polymyositis and dermatomyositis: widespread inflammatory disease, with weakness of muscles, primarily of the shoulders, pelvis, and neck.

    Symptoms: Pain and weakness in muscles, tenderness, difficulty in standing up, climbing stairs, reaching high over head. With dermatomyositis a red rash usually erupts on the face, neck, upper back, chest, and arms. Rash on eyelids accompanied by swelling around the eyes.

    Cause: Unknown.

    Treatment: Anti-inflammatory drugs.

So, here are ten debilitating, painful immune disorders. Notice anything striking about them? How could you not? It would be easier to miss a kangaroo in your living room than to miss the similarities with them. It's as though I'm using ten different names to describe the exact same thing. Remember, rain, ice, snow, sleet, and hail are all the same thing—water in different states of consistency. Lupus, fibromyalgia, chronic fatigue syndrome, rheumatoid arthritis are also all the same thing—toxins that have overwhelmed the lymph system.

Do you recall the five most universal and obvious symptoms of a lymph system in distress? Pain, fatigue, irregular sleep, loss of appetite, and fever. They're all here! Do you further recall that the fourth stage—inflammation—is the stage where there's lots of pain and discomfort and is the point in the disease process at which you had better do something to support your lymph system's efforts to cleanse itself or you're begging for it? Eight of these ten list inflammation as a symptom. Half are treated with anti-inflammatories. So many anti-inflammatories are being prescribed that the inevitable was bound to occur: with greater regularity, it is being reported that anti-inflammatories are causing negative side effects, including osteoporosis and bleeding stomach ulcers. Trading one disease for another.

To anyone even remotely aware of the nature of the lymph system, how it operates, and what it does, nothing could be more obvious. And yet all are, according to the experts, mysterious ailments without explanation. With all ten, the cause is supposedly unknown. With all ten, drugs are the treatment. Yet to drug the body so as to mask the pain, without removing the cause of the pain, guarantees that the disease state will inevitably progress to the next stage of disease.

Now, I am not minimizing the seriousness of these immune disorders. Far too many people have suffered or are presently suffering with them for me to do that. But whether we're talking about the ones I've listed or others such as asthma, allergies, hives, or any of a few lesser known immune disorders, the diligent use of the CARE principles will not only prevent them from developing, but will also bring relief to anyone presently dealing with them, and in many cases reverse them entirely.

CARDIOVASCULAR (HEART AND BLOOD VESSEL) DISORDERS

Cardiovascular disease is the biggest killer in this country, taking more lives than all other diseases combined. With conscientious effort, cardiovascular disease can definitely be avoided. The works of Nathan Pritikin, Julian Whitaker, M.D., Dean Ornish, M.D., and others have certainly proved that to be so. I want to focus here on just two important aspects of the disease and show how they are affected by the proper care and treatment of the lymph system.

HIGH BLOOD PRESSURE

Also known as hypertension, high blood pressure exerts too much pressure against the walls of the arteries. This can damage the heart with a heart attack, the brain with a stroke, the retina to the point of blindness, and the kidneys to the point of failure. We are told that in most people the cause is unknown. The treatment for it is, you guessed it, drugs. Yet according to Dr. Herbert Shelton, the father of Natural Hygiene, "Perhaps the single greatest cause of high blood pressure is toxemia resulting from checked elimination." If wastes (toxins) build in the body beyond the lymph system's ability to eliminate them, they will cause trouble, whether in an organ, or on the skin, or in the delicate arteries and blood vessels of the cardiovascular system. It doesn't matter where, only that it happened.

I have a great deal of experience with high blood pressure in people. I have seen, more times than I can recount, people who completely overcame high blood pressure by properly caring for the lymph system. One of my older brothers (not the one who stole my fried chicken thigh) was on high blood pressure medication for ten years without ever having his blood pressure be in the normal range. After diligently using the CARE principles to cleanse his lymph system, his blood pressure went to normal for the first time in ten years and stayed there, with no drugs. This was over twelve years ago.

A note of caution here: When you start the CARE principles to normalize your blood pressure, do not, I repeat, do not stop your medication abruptly. As you start to clean your system of wastes and relieve the pressure on your arteries, you must gradually reduce the drugs and have your pressure checked regularly.

HEART ATTACK

A heart attack occurs when one of the heart's arteries fails to deliver enough blood to the part of the heart muscle it serves. I don't know from experience, thank goodness, but people who have described the persistent, crushing chest pain that can spread to the left arm, jaw, neck or shoulder blades, as akin to having a piano dropped on you. It's something even the most curious of the curious would not want to experience first-hand.

The primary cause of heart attack is arteriosclerosis, the hardening or thickening of the artery wall which causes loss of elasticity. The second most common cause is atherosclerosis, the condition in which the arteries become so packed with fat and cholesterol that the blood can't flow. As discussed in Chapter Five, one of the primary functions of the lymph system is to remove fat from the digestive tract before it can ever reach your arteries. In other words, when the lymph system is functioning properly, the arteries carrying the river of life through your body are kept clean and supple. That is its job.

If your lymph system is not overburdened with unelimi-nated wastes and is operating efficiently, the chances of you developing cardiovascular disease of any kind is, in my opinion, too small to calculate. Cardiovascular disease and cells that have been driven crazy represent the two biggest killers the world has ever known. Between them, over 4,000 people die every single day! Yet they are both entirely pre-ventable. You can live your life with the absolute knowledge that you will never have to deal personally with either. The deep, priceless feeling of contentment and security that comes with that knowledge is yours for the asking. Taking proper care of your lymph system and reaping the rewards cost you nothing. Your body does it for you for free if you give it the opportunity. It will, in the long run, save you money. And some might say that that is the very reason you have not heard anything about it until now.

DIGESTIVE DISORDERS

The seventy tons of food we eat in a lifetime and the effect it has on the digestive tract has been my area of interest and study for 30 years. I'm telling you, I hardly know where to begin here. I could write a book on this subject alone. The digestive tract, or alimentary canal, is thirty feet long, starting at your mouth and ending where wastes find their way to the outside world. All along the way there are twists and turns, wrinkles and folds, cracks and crevices, nooks and crannies, corners and pockets galore. Lots of places where uneliminated wastes can accumulate, stagnate, and become inflamed if not removed. If you look over the list of possible digestive disorders, of which there are dozens, there are lots of names ending in -*itis*. You know what that means: inflammation; the fourth stage of disease; lots of pain and discomfort; and as the symptoms of the supposedly different maladies are perused, the word "inflammation" is as commonplace as feathers on a duck.

It's a sad commentary indeed that the true nature of inflammation is not understood by traditional medicine. Rather than being acknowledged as the result of uneliminated toxins that have been in the body for far too long, it is instead blamed on a most reliable scapegoat: viral or bacterial infection. It's so easy to blame an enemy that we can't see, so we don't have to take any responsibility for the situation. Of course, there will be large numbers of bacteria in the gut of a toxic individual, but the bacteria is not the *cause* of the disorder. No more than flies are the cause of the garbage they can invariably be found feeding upon. If you saw a pile of garbage with flies buzzing all around it, would you say, "Look at all that garbage those flies have dragged in here?" To blame inflammation on the bacteria that happen to be feeding on the toxins causing the inflammation is the same as blaming garbage on flies.

I'm going to use four recognizable disorders of the digestive tract to illustrate the role the lymph system plays. There are plenty more including esophagitis, diverticulitis, gastroenteritis, gastritis, irritable bowel syndrome, pancreatitis, peritonitis, and others.

COLITIS

The word "colitis" means inflammation of the colon, but by now, you knew that, didn't you? Let's take a look at how traditional medicine views colitis, which is an inflammatory, often chronic disease that affects the lining of the lower intestine. It starts in the lowest section (where feces are held until evacuated) and often extends upward into the colon, producing swelling and sometimes open sores. If open sores are present, it is referred to as ulcerative colitis. The primary symptoms are repeated attacks of pain, the intensity of which varies with the extent of inflammation, irritability, bloody diarrhea, loss of appetite, weakness, and nausea. We are told that the exact cause of colitis is unknown, but that it is possibly associated with a bacteria of some kind. And of course, it is treated with, antiinflammatory drugs. This will mask the pain so the disease process can continue until cells are ultimately driven crazy.

Everything You Need to Know About Diseases, a wonderful book written by over one hundred leading doctors and medical experts, states, "People with colitis run a higher than average risk of developing cancer, especially if the disease persists, for longer than 10 years."[106] Excuse me, while I loudly clear my throat. This is precisely my point. If inflammation is allowed to persist by dulling the pain with drugs, eventually, as you learned earlier, the nonstop assault of toxins on the cells will drive them crazy. Support the lymph system's natural attempt to cleanse the inflammatory toxins from the system and pain stops, the disease process stops, and cells are not driven crazy. It's that simple.

CROHN'S DISEASE

This is described as inflammation of any part of the digestive system. Well, if that's the case, why isn't colitis, which is inflammation of the lower intestines, also called Crohn's? The lower intestines are part of the digestive system, aren't they? These are not two different diseases. And guess what? Another disease called enteritis is defined as inflammation of the intestines especially of the lower intestine. So how is enteritis differentiated from colitis or Crohn's? There is no difference! The symptoms of Crohn's are pain, fatigue, fever, diarrhea, etc. Treatment is . . . anti-inflammatory drugs. When Crohn's flares up, it is said to mimic appendicitis, which we'll get to shortly.

One doctor noted that "colitis, Crohn's, and enteritis are all inflammatory conditions causing damage to the intestinal lining. You can have severe inflammation in the lower intestine and call it Crohn's or enteritis, and half an inch away in the colon it's called colitis." The cause of Crohn's, in any case, is "unknown."

PEPTIC ULCERS

These are open sores that develop in the lining of the stomach and sections of the intestines. Ulcers represent the fifth stage of disease—ulceration—when the body simply can hold out no longer against the long-term assault of toxins and inflammation so a sore opens up. The symptoms are pain, pain, and more pain. The cause is not known and the treatment is antiinflammatory drugs. (You must be getting as tired of reading this over and over as I am of writing it.)

APPENDICITIS

I saved this particular "itis" for last for a very good reason. It's the crowning example of the ignorance traditional medicine has of the true nature of inflammation in the human body.

Once again, we're being asked to accept the absurd notion that the Grand Creator of all and everything actually placed in one of the most complex, infinitely intelligent life forms on this planet a worthless organ with no purpose other than to cause grief. Past members of this elite club, of course, include the tonsils.

For a hundred years, natural hygienists have been battling the powers that be over their obstinate belief that the tonsils and appendix are worthless and expendable. It's gratifying that the tonsils are now more frequently allowed to stay where God put them, but, alas, the appendix has yet to be similarly pardoned.

We are told that appendicitis is a medical emergency in which the appendix is inflamed due to a blockage of the lymph system. This obstruction "may" be caused by a bit of uneliminated waste or a viral infection. Symptoms include pain in or around the lower right abdomen, loss of appetite, nausea, constipation or diarrhea, slight fever, and tenderness to the touch near the area of the abdomen. Standard medical treatment is antibiotics and bedrest and, if the appendix remains inflamed, to cut it out and throw it away with a "good riddance." Yet as one doctor notes, "There *are* cases in which appendicitis, particularly when it has been undiagnosed for some time, requires surgical intervention, but those cases are relatively few. There are many adjuvant therapies, such as diet and enzymatic therapy, that can prevent it from progressing to that point."

In numerous books on physiology that I have looked at, the only discussion of the appendix is about the misery it brings. Only in one did I actually ever find a reference to what its function might be: "none in man so far as is known."[107]

Now, let's take a look at the nonfiction version. The version that honors and respects the unfathomable wisdom, intelligence, and grandeur of the human body. The version that reveres the dynamics of the body knowing that it was created in magnificent harmony, with no "extra" parts that are unnecessary, but rather with the ability to repair, heal, and maintain itself with a precision unknown in our highly technological age.

Remember, the alimentary canal is thirty feet long in total. The small intestine is about twenty-two feet long. *Small* here isn't describing its length, but rather is circumference. It empties into the large intestine, which is about five feet long but much wider in circumference. The large intestine is also referred to as the colon.

After all the processes of metabolism have been performed and everything the body needs from food has been extracted, the waste is held in the colon before elimination. This fecal matter is highly toxic and needs to be removed from the body as quickly and efficiently as possible. The last thing you want is for any of this toxic, fecal matter to stay in the body, where it can inflame and cause harm. Forced to stay in the body, it can impact itself in the lining of the colon causing great discomfort. Crohn's, colitis, and irritable bowel are all the result of uneliminated waste that became impacted and inflamed. The appendix is strategically placed at the highest part of the colon, right where the small intestine empties into it. What few people understand is that the appendix generates and secretes a powerful substance to neutralize and remove any residue from the colon that may become impacted and inflamed. Considering the immense intelligence of the human body, doesn't that make a heck of a lot more sense than saying the appendix is a mistake of nature?

In case you think I'm making this up, consider that I learned of this from one of the most respected and revered nutritional scientists the world has ever known: Dr. Norman W. Walker, who wrote at least six books that I know of and passed away peacefully and healthfully in his sleep at age 106. He was health personified and knew full well that the appendix, like every other part of the magnificent human body, has purpose and is right where it's supposed to be.

I learned of the true function of the appendix in 1970 and since that time I have been inquiring from anyone who has had a particularly hard time losing weight if they had their appendix. Invariably, those people who had weight problems to begin with and who had lost their appendix all told me that losing weight became even more of an ordeal since the loss of their appendix.

If that describes you, don't worry, all is not lost. What it does mean however, is that you, more so than those who still have their appendix intact, have to be particularly diligent with the CARE principles.

Traditional medicine views inflammation as an enemy, the cause of which is rarely known but which must be attacked and subdued at all costs. Natural Hygiene views inflammation as a friendly but stern warning from the body that uneliminated toxins have reached a critical level.

One of the worst possible actions you can take when the inflammatory stage of disease develops (fourth stage) is to go to battle against it with drugs. Not only do the drugs hide the fact from you that the lymph system is struggling with wastes to the point where tissue is becoming inflamed, but also the drugs, all of which are toxic and have side effects of their own, add more toxins to the already overburdened lymph system. Drugs in this instance can only make things worse.

One of the anti-inflammatory drugs prescribed for lupus was reported on CNN News to cause the premature aging of bones, resulting in osteoporosis. On the ABC news program "20/20" it was reported that anti-inflammatory drugs cause bleeding stomach ulcers. Trading one disease for another disease can hardly be classified as health care. I have said it before, and I'll say it some more: you can't poison yourself back to health. Get away from that way of thinking. Do the right thing for your body and it will reward you in kind many times over.

The biggest killer of all time is cardiovascular disease. I have shown you how the proper care and treatment of the lymph system will protect you from this scourge. The second biggest killer is cancer. I have shown you how this can be prevented as well by the same effort to keep the lymph system clean. The same is true for autoimmune diseases and digestive disorders. Here again, you now know how to prevent them as well through properly CAREing for your lymph system.

At first glance, cardiovascular disease, cancer, immune disorders, and digestive tract disorders appear to be four widely divergent maladies. Nonetheless, the same measures to prevent one will prevent all four. Now, I could keep on going and discuss lung and breathing disorders, nervous system disorders, muscle and bone disorders, liver and gall bladder disorders, kidney and urinary disorders, skin disorders, and on and on. But what would be the point? The remedy is the same. How many times do you have to hear that the cause is unknown but there's a drug to mask its symptoms?

Perhaps I have not specifically mentioned whatever health problem you may be concerned with, but simply transpose it with any of the ones I have mentioned because I would be recommending the same course of action: *Clean your lymph system!* And instead of saying something to the effect of, "How could it possibly be so simple?" say instead, "How marvelously freeing it is for it to actually be so simple." Just because the people who "don't know" think it's so very much more complicated than it actually is doesn't make it so.

The unassailable fact is that your lymph system is the mechanism in the body designed *specifically* to keep you well and keep you alive. You take CARE of it, it will take care of you. You will find this out for yourself as so many others have done before you. The human body is so quick to respond to proper care that some measure of improvement will manifest itself almost immediately.

What is your alternative? What is your alternative to assisting and supporting your body in functioning as efficiently and effectively as possible? It is to fall into the pharmaceutical industry's web of drugs.

We've already learned that over 2 million people are seriously injured, and 106,000 die every year, from the *correct* use of prescription drugs. But what is even more alarming is that, by all accounts, the situation is, as you are reading this, becoming much, much worse. Why? Because rather than putting measures in place to have some safeguards to protect the public, FDA officials are instead resigned to the danger growing because they are now approving new drugs at a record pace.[108]

According to Dr. Kenneth Kizer, Undersecretary for Health at the Department of Veteran's Affairs in Washington, "There are so many new drugs available, that keeping current with the information that goes with each drug has become almost impossible."[109] Regulators cannot even predict all the potential side effects or toxic reactions. According to an article in the *New York Times,* "The true scope of the problem is unknown, in part because hospitals and doctors are not required to report it."[110]

Injuries and deaths, as abominably high as they are today, are going to increase, and everybody involved knows it. In the words of Dr. Lucian Leape, a health policy analyst at the Harvard School of Public Health, "Adverse drug events are a disease of medical progress."[111] So if your spouse or your child or your father or mother drops dead from a prescription, they've had an "adverse drug event."

There is a nonprofit consumer advocacy organization on your side that investigates "adverse drug events." Michael Cohen, president of the Institute for Safe Medication Practices, says that, "the technology to prevent patient harm has not been developed, and the resources are not being invested to protect patients."[112] Guess why? It's too expensive!

In 1992 there were 2.03 billion prescriptions dispensed. In 1998 it rose to 2.78 billion. And in 2005 it will be 4 billion. But it's already out of control *now.* There are *already* no means to determine what harm the toxic side effects can cause. There are *already* no safeguards to protect you. There are *already* more than 100,000 people dying every year. And the only action being taken for sure is to dramatically *increase* the number of drugs being approved. It's insanity. Truly. What would you call it? If someone were drowning in a pool, do you think that adding water to the pool would help?

You owe it to yourself and those you love to pay attention to what I'm saying here. Protect yourself. The drug industry sure won't. Clean your lymph system to prevent the need for drugs and you won't run the risk of suffering from an "adverse drug event."

The idea that I'm presenting—that most disease has a single cause and a single remedy—is going to be difficult for some to accept. I know that. And I am fully aware of the fact that I'm challenging the institutions, dominant beliefs, and the authority figures of our culture. The same way the Wright Brothers did when they said, "Oh yeah? We can too fly!"

Whenever a certain philosophy makes dramatic proclamations in opposition to prevailing thought, detractors will try to find a chink in the armor—exceptions that destroy the premise being offered up. Let me be the first to say there will be exceptions to what I'm telling you. Cleaning one's lymph system will not prevent all disease. Just as an example, if someone eats a low-fiber, calcium-poor diet, dominated by a lot of protein foods which leach calcium from the bones, that person has an extremely high chance of developing osteoporosis, irrespective of the cleanliness or efficiency of his or her lymph system.

There are simply too many variables that contribute to how and why people become sick. Plus, there is far more about the human body and how it works that we don't know than we do know. Even under the best of circumstances, even when people live well and keep their lymph systems clean and healthy, sickness can still occur. Perhaps an inherited genetic weakness causes an organ to fail. Or perhaps some other group of factors of which no one is even aware leads to some malady. We are dealing with an immensely complex subject that is literally in its embryonic stages of being understood. No one—not me, not anyone—can legitimately make a universal, blanket statement about how and why the human body does what it does. Quite frankly, guesswork, speculation, and educated predictions based on past evidence are about the best that can be expected.

So, I want you to be unquestionably clear that I am not suggesting that following the recommendations in this book guarantees uninterrupted, vibrant health for everyone who does so. Of the approximately 2,000,000 deaths by disease each year in this country, what if a third were to somehow be prevented? Such an event would go down in history as one of the greatest advances the world has ever known. Well, after the many years of firsthand experience I have had, in my heart of hearts, I know that if every person in the United States were to diligently follow the recommendations in this book, closer to 80 percent or more of all diseases would be prevented. As one doctor states, "There is no question that detoxification can decrease one's risk of dying from organ system failure. Toxins block and poison many enzymes which control cell energy cycles, immunity, the production of antiaging hormones, and many life-saving functions of the body."[113]

I just wish to acknowledge to you that I understand what a daunting challenge it is to read a single book with such dramatic, revolutionary ideas and then simply accept them as gospel. That's not how it works. People have to live with the principles, use them, and see over time if their health is steadily improving or not. My biggest question to you is this: What if I'm right? What exactly do you have to lose by ensuring that the mechanism in your body in charge of keeping you well and keeping you alive is clean and in optimum working condition? There is one guarantee I'll make to you without the slightest degree of hesitation. You will never, ever see in an obituary column a cause of death being attributed to insufficient toxins in the lymphatic system.

EIGHT

Too Fat or Not Too Fat

I love to eat. I love food and I love to eat. Always have, too. I think the opening of the book established that. I love everything about food. I enjoy thinking about it, looking at it, talking about it, preparing it, smelling it, tasting it, and eating it. Going to a new restaurant and sampling its cuisine is as exciting an adventure for me as going to a thrilling sports event may be for someone else. So I am not the least bit surprised that my life revolves around the study and teaching of the effect of nutrition on the human body. I don't mind telling you that I feel blessed to have been given the ability to grasp the important relationship between nutrition and good health. Frankly, had I not grasped the concept, considering the road I was on, I would probably be dead or as close to it as one can be and still be breathing.

In terms of my health, the difference between the first twenty-five years of my life and the second twenty-five years is like the difference between a barren strip-mine site and a lush rain forest. My first twenty-five years of life was an

ongoing battle against pain, excess weight, and lethargy. I suffered from excruciating stomach pains, frequent headaches,
including migraines, numerous colds and sinus problems, a
perennial lack of energy, and ultimately reached a weight of over
200 pounds. This sorry situation occurred because my love for
eating knew no bounds. I was never raised with or taught anything about the effect of food on my health. My only prerequisite for what I would eat was, could I get it down my throat?

In 1970, at age twenty-five, I had the immeasurable good
fortune to be introduced to Natural Hygiene, and since that
time, I have had no stomachaches, headaches, or sinus problems. I have an abundance of energy and the 50 pounds I
quickly lost have stayed off. And the really good news, for me
anyway, is that I achieved all this while still reveling in the
joys of eating. The difference is, I learned how to fully enjoy
the eating experience and maintain my health.

NUTRITION AND VIBRANT HEALTH

There are many factors involved in the development of
disease, be it cells that are driven crazy or any other illness.
The most prominent are: the quality of our food, air, and water;
exercise; rest and sleep; sunshine; loving relationships; self-
love and inner peace; and our mental processes. I know that all
of these variables, and more, play a role in whether or not we
become ill, but I am certain beyond any possible doubt that far
and away the Number 1 factor affecting our health and well-
being is the food and water we consume. This is a conviction
based on my own extensive experience and on both mine and
others' observations.

A biochemist and certified nutritionist who is the director of
a well-known chronic disease treatment facility, has this to say:

"The latest research utilizing PCR (polymerase chain reaction) testing is an amazing breakthrough in identifying the
unsuspected role of infection in causing chronic diseases rang-

ing from Alzheimer's to heart disease to cancer. However, infection is only possible when there is a pronounced nutritional deficiency.

"The increasing chemical exposure that we receive from our air, water, and food, coupled with foods that have been irradiated, microwaved, or grown from hybrid seeds or seeds that have been genetically altered, all dramatically increase the body's demand for nutrients in an effort to detoxify these multiple toxic agents. Repeated daily exposure to these toxins can waste the body's stores of nutrients very rapidly, leading to rampant nutritional deficiencies.

"Once the body has become deficient, the stage has been set for infection to take place; as the nutritional deficiency persists over time, the infection fostered can become chronic. Now merely correcting the deficiency may not be enough to eliminate the infection. Worse yet, chronic infection can create hormone deficiencies or immune system imbalances, which in turn lock in the infection, leaving you in a downward spiral of ever-increasing immune burden, fatigue and accelerated aging."

If we were to rate all foods that we consume, obviously something would have to be ranked the very best food for our health and something would have to be the most detrimental, with everything else falling somewhere in between. Later on I'm going to talk about the very best, but right now it is essential that I talk about the one at the other end of the scale: food which, if eaten in excess, will do more to increase your chances of developing ill health than any other.

ANIMAL PRODUCTS

The greatest threat to your health is the overconsumption of animal products. Animal products include all meat, chicken, fish, eggs, and dairy products. I am convinced that the overconsumption of them is the leading cause of a clogged lymph system, excess weight, pain, ill health, disease, suffering, and death.

Of course, these are words that anger organizations like the cattlemen's association and the dairy council. After all, the animal products industries take in over a quarter of a trillion dollars a year; so they hardly want you to find out the truth about their products. One major strategy they use is to call out their hired "experts" to scare the blood out of the veins of anyone who would even contemplate investigating a diet that contains little or no animal products. The people making the trillions of dollars selling animal products would have you believe that the next three generations of your descendants will be condemned to all manner of deficiencies and disease if you skip meat or milk at even one meal. A slight exaggeration, but they do get a bit carried away when our quest for health starts to interfere with their profits.

Actually, their attempts to dissuade us from eating less of their products are becoming increasingly more difficult because of the vast amount of data consistently coming forth that proves our love affair with animal products has been and remains a major contributor to ill health. To clarify my position and head off any campaign by the animal products industries to label me as something I'm not, I wish to spell out precisely where I stand in relation to the "V" word.

VEGETARIANISM

Vegetarianism is ideally the healthiest way to eat, but vegetarianism is not for everyone. I know vegetarians who have had their lives saved by eliminating meat and dairy from their diet. I also know strict vegetarians whose health suffered until they reintroduced some animal products into their diets. Anyone who insists that vegetarianism is the only truly healthy way to eat is just as off base as someone who insists you can't be truly healthy if you are a vegetarian.

Being a vegetarian is an exceedingly personal choice and depends on many variables that relate to each individual's characteristics and unique circumstances. Just because a vegetarian diet works well for some people does not automatically mean it will work for everyone. It is as objectionable to demand that people embrace vegetarianism as it would be to tell them to change religions. There are those who understand intellectually that cutting meat and dairy from their diets is best, but because they were raised on those foods and have eaten them for years, they're up against a tremendous amount of physical and emotional conditioning.

There is, however, something that everyone can do, and that many people are already doing, to take advantage of the most up-to-date research on the subject: Cut back! For decades we have been overeating animal products. Research on the effect of this overconsumption is overwhelmingly conclusive: It is killing us!

In *Fit for Life*, and especially in *Fit for Life II*, I discussed in great detail the full extent to which animal products contribute to every major disease. I challenged several dietary myths: the four food group mentality; the daily need for huge amounts of protein; the idea that meat is the best source of protein; and the notion that dairy was essential for calcium intake and for protection against osteoporosis.

Today, it is no longer a matter of debate whether we should reduce our intake of animal products, but solely on the extent to which we should reduce it. Opinions range from a conservative cutback of 15 percent or 20 percent to total abstinence from all animal products. What you as a person motivated to achieve vibrant health must decide is what extent would be most comfortable and work best in your life. One thing is certain: Lowering your intake of animal products is going to have a beneficial effect on your health commensurate with the extent to which you reduce these foods in your diet.

Let's look at why.

THE KILLERS—CHOLESTEROL AND FAT

Do the words "cholesterol" and "saturated fat" sound familiar? Twenty years ago, you hardly, if ever, heard these terms. Today it is nearly impossible to go through a single day without hearing or reading something about them, and with good reason. They kill people! Lots of people. In fact, the argument is very strong that, together, cholesterol and fat kill more people than any other single cause of death in the United States.

Where do these killers come from? Absolutely all cholesterol comes from animal products. Cholesterol is produced in the liver and cells of animals (including humans) and nowhere else. It is impossible to ingest cholesterol from the plant kingdom.

If you have any concern or problem with cholesterol, it is the result of the animal foods in your diet. Reduce them and you reduce your level of cholesterol. A simple formula. Yet people still get confused about this. They will ask, "What about avocados, nuts, and oils? Don't they contain cholesterol?" Since none of these have a liver, they contain no cholesterol.

What these people are doing is confusing cholesterol with fat, which is found in *all* foods. However, the vast, vast majority of fat, including saturated fats, comes from animal products as well. And although cholesterol is an important contributing factor to ill health, it is now well understood that fat in the American diet is as much or more of a cause for concern.

SATURATED FATS AND HEART DISEASE

As we have seen, cardiovascular disease, which includes heart disease, all atherosclerotic diseases of the blood vessels, and stroke, kills more people than all other causes of death combined![114]* It kills nearly one million people a year, two and a half thousand every day! When blood is constricted and unable to get to the heart, a heart attack is the result. When the blood is prevented from reaching the brain, a stroke or "heart attack of the brain" occurs.

What causes the veins to be blocked? Plaque. What is plaque? A thick coating of cholesterol and fat trapped in the arteries which the body has been unable to remove. And you can be sure that if these substances are overburdening the cardiovascular system, they are doing the same to the lymph system, as you will see shortly. Certainly many other factors contribute to cardiovascular disease, and animal products are not the exclusive cause, but they are unquestionably the major cause. The abundance of research corroborating the direct link between fat and cholesterol levels and heart disease is irrefutable. It is the leading predictor of atherosclerosis (clogged arteries) and subsequent heart disease.[115]

Dr. Marc Sorenson, the author of three highly comprehensive and informative books and founder of the National Institute of Fitness in Ivins, Utah, where thousands of people from all over the world go to recapture their health, has this to say on the subject of heart disease:

Heart disease is an insidious and unnecessary malady which is caused explicitly by the consumption of animal

---

*You already have learned that cells being driven crazy (cancer) is the second biggest killer, with lung cancer leading all other types. Obviously, this is because of smoking.

It's been my experience that people who smoke also indulge in dietary indiscretions that contribute to their ill health. By the way, a study conducted by the American Cancer Society on more than 600,000 women concluded that smoking escalates a woman's risk of dying from breast cancer by at least 25 percent. The more cigarettes a woman smokes and the longer she smokes, the greater the risk. The study also said that the risk is eliminated by quitting.121

products and saturated fat. It is predictable, preventable, reversible, and wholly unnecessary.[116]

And yet about 1 in 4 Americans die from heart disease,[117] while $12 billion are spent annually on bypass sur-gery,[118] which is actually worse than doing nothing![119] What is imperative for you to know and never lose sight of is that while animal proteins definitely raise cholesterol levels, vegetable protein can reduce them![120]

THE CASE AGAINST ANIMAL PRODUCTS

Whenever I attempt to impart information that may be new for some people, I have always asked them to rely as much on their common sense as on the so-called "scientific proof." Because, frankly, under the right circumstances and with proper funding, scientists can "prove" anything they want. Medical libraries are rife with examples of "scientific studies" that have proved one premise only to be replaced by other studies that prove the opposite.

I already gave you the example earlier of the two studies in the same journal "proving" estrogen both prevents and causes heart disease. As another quick example, consider the "incredible edible egg." There is certainly nothing wrong with eating eggs on occasion, but they do contain one of the highest concentrations of cholesterol of any food. Data abounds showing this to be so. Eggs are the choice of researchers when they want to study their subjects' staggering increases in cholesterol levels.[122] In fact, eggs will increase blood cholesterol levels more effectively than pure cholesterol dissolved in oil![123] Yet five studies "prove," of all things, that eggs do not raise blood cholesterol levels.[124] The five studies, by the way, just happened to be funded by the egg industry.[125]

These examples demonstrate why it is so difficult to rely solely on scientific studies and scientific experts, and why observation and common sense have to be given equal weight when making decisions about what actions you're going to take on your own behalf. This is particularly important with regard to fat as a major risk factor in cancer. There is at present a controversy raging in the scientific community about this very subject. Once again, the "experts" are divided; half think there is conclusive evidence and half think there is inconclusive evidence. How this can be absolutely boggles my mind. To me, there is about as much doubt that fat is indeed a risk factor in driving cells crazy as there is doubt that the world is round, not flat. I will do my best to prove this to you using both scientific data and common sense.

REDUCE THE FAT NOW!

Those who are convinced that fat is a risk factor feel that there is sufficient evidence incriminating fat to reduce intake of it now. Those who are not convinced agree that there is evidence pointing to fat as a possible villain, but since there are no studies that absolutely and definitively prove that to be so, they want more research to be conducted before they can feel certain that it is so and make recommendations accordingly. Since I am one of those for whom no further proof is needed, I am going to give you all the reasons I think you should reduce your fat intake now. Then you can decide for yourself.

In October 1988, the Surgeon General's Report on Health and Nutrition exploded on the front page of newspapers all over the country. After reviewing more than 2,500 scientific studies on the subject, the nation's top medical doctor removed any hope the animal products industry might have had of not being incriminated. In the report, and in interview after interview, the message from the Surgeon General was clear: Cholesterol and fat (animal products) are wreaking havoc on the nation's health. His advice: Cut back on these foods and add more fiber to your diet in the form of fruits, vegetables, whole grains, and legumes. Although he did not label them as such, these, of course, are the cleansing foods.

Then the National Institutes of Health released their recommendations. Same again. Plus there were the recommendations of the Senate Select Committee on Nutrition and Human Needs in 1977, the American Heart Association in 1979, the National Cancer Institute in 1979, the American Cancer Society in 1984, and at least twenty other authoritative agencies and organizations in the United States and abroad. All said the same thing: Animal products are wreaking havoc on the nation's health.

Right behind lung cancer, colon cancer is the second leading cause of cancer deaths. In 1990, two major studies were published that dealt with diet and colon cancer. Both looked at large numbers of people over a long period of time. Both studies reached similar conclusions. They indicated meat eating as a major risk factor in colon cancer.[126] One of the studies reported in the *New England Journal of Medicine* followed more than 88,000 subjects for six years. Its findings indicated that the more animal fat eaten, the more likely it was that colon cancer would result. Those eating the most animal fat were nearly twice as likely to develop colon cancer as those eating the least animal fat.

Dr. Walter Willet, who directed the study, concluded: "If you step back and look at the data, the optimum amount of red meat you eat should be zero."[127] Typical of the research I see, this study made no mention of the importance of cleansing the colon, the most effective measure an individual can take to prevent all cancers, including that of the colon. Animal products, which are very high in cholesterol and fat and devoid of fiber, serve only to block and toxify the colon. High-fiber plant foods (all fruits, vegetables, and grains) are the colon's best protection against cancer. It is noteworthy that women who consume the highest amount of vegetables have one-tenth the rate of breast cancer as those who eat the least amount.[128]

In 1989, the Surgeon General's report was followed up by recommendations from the National Academy of Sciences. After taking three years to review 6,000 research studies, the academy released what it called the "most definitive dietary recommendations in the history of the organization."[129] It was the Surgeon General's recommendations all over again.

When you have that kind of unanimity among top authorities, it's time to pay attention. For so many in the medical community to now so strongly and so unanimously concur with the very findings they denied as recently as the late 1980s sends the clearest possible message: The amount of evidence supporting the recommendation to reduce our intake of animal products has to be titanic. And when they finally link the case for reducing animal products with the individual's ability to prevent illness by cleansing the body, they will have the whole picture and we will begin to enjoy an approach to health care that is truly grounded in prevention.

There are numerous studies that make a compelling correlation between breast cancer and the consumption of dietary fat.[130] And fat intake also has an impact on a couple of the other suspected risk factors. One of those suspected risk factors is the female sex hormone estrogen. According to *Science News,* "Scientists don't understand exactly how estrogen fosters breast cancer[131] but the consensus is that the more estrogen there is in the blood, the more likelihood of developing breast cancer. High-fat diets cause high levels of estrogen in women.[132] Comparisons reveal that women who eat meat have significantly higher levels of estrogen in their blood than vegetarian women.[133] And when women switch to low-fat diets, the levels of estrogen drop sharply.[134]

Another suspected risk factor in developing breast cancer is late menopause. A correlation has been shown between late menopause and excessive fat in the diet.[135]

One very convincing piece of evidence incriminating dietary fat as a risk factor that promotes breast cancer is the well-documented rise of breast cancer in Japanese women who either come to North America and change their diet or stay home and change their traditional diet (plant-based) to a North American diet (animal-based). An article in the *FDA Consumer* states that, "The death rate from breast cancer is the highest in countries like the United States, where the intake of fat and animal protein is high."[136] Further, it commented that Japanese women historically have a low risk for breast cancer, but that risk has been rising dramatically, concurrent with a "westernization" of eating habits, that is, from a low-fat to high-fat diet. Other research that has studied fat consumption of women living in Japan or Japanese women who come to the United States and increase their fat intake also confirms that the more fat eaten, the higher the incidence of breast cancer in these women.[137] An article in *Newsweek* commented on the hazard of a western diet (beef, dairy, and other fat-laden foods)

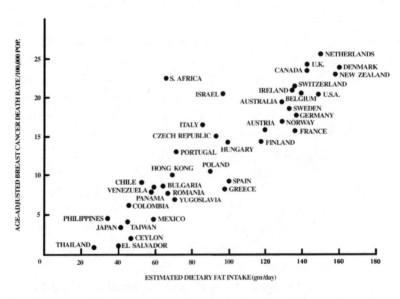

Relationship of Dietary Fat Consumption to Death from Breast Cancer

to Japanese women. The article was titled "Death by Fried Chicken."[138]

Japanese women are not alone in this. The chart below illustrates clearly the correlation between fat intake and breast cancer in various countries. It is no accident that the incidence of breast cancer increases commensurately with the increase in fat consumption.

Researchers at the National Cancer Institute reanalyzed 100 animal experiments pertaining to fats, calories, and cancer, and concluded that each excess fat-derived calorie posed 67 percent more risk than calories from other sources. A study of Finnish women found that the participants who later developed cancer showed a "consistently higher" average percent of fat-derived calories.[139]

THE GLORIOUS PLANT-RICH DIET

As important as it is to become aware of the foods, such as animal products, that put you at risk of cancer, it is every bit as important to know what foods contain compounds capable of retarding cancer. The more researchers understand about the ingredients in fruits, vegetables, and other plant-based foods, the more impressed they are with the power of these compounds to retard the bodily breakdown that results in driving cells crazy. Consider the following comment from an editorial in the *New York Times:* "Nutritionists and epidemiologists have long observed that people who eat a plant rich diet suffer lower rates of cancer than do meat loyalists."[140]

I guarantee that you will not see headlines proclaiming that some special ingredient in a pork chop or a hamburger has been isolated and has been found to fight cancer. The helpful constituents of food that are becoming increasingly familiar all come from plant foods, not animal foods. Compounds like flavonoids, carotenes, phytonutrients, antioxidants, fiber, and many,

many more are all derived from plant foods. Every time you hear about some newly discovered multisyllabic compound that fights disease, it is derived from fruits, vegetables, grains, or some other plant food.

No doubt you have heard mention of free radicals and antioxidants. Let's see if I can give you a simple, easily understood explanation of them. Body cells make use of oxygen in breaking down proteins, fats, and carbohydrates. In the process, free radicals are formed. These oxygen molecules undermine the orderly process of cell life by careening around your body looking for what they need to survive, and in so doing, damage healthy cells. Many authorities are convinced that free radicals kick off the cancer process. All agree that free radicals are a danger.

Dr. Keith Block, Medical Director of the Cancer Institute at Edgewater Hospital in Chicago, says, "A high fat diet steps up the body's production of free radicals, which increase damage to the body's genetic material."[141] Cells protect themselves with compounds called antioxidants, which are the policemen, if you will, that subdue free radicals. Fruits and vegetables are packed with antioxidants that either stop the formation of free radicals, or disable them before they do harm. *High-fat animal products stimulate the development of free radicals. Antioxidant rich fruits and vegetables prevent their formation.*

Have you heard of sulforaphane? Its discovery resulted in a headline that read, BROCCOLI EXTRACT SHOWN TO BLOCK BREAST CANCER.[142] Researchers at Johns Hopkins University made the discovery and reported it to the media. Sulforaphane is a substance that is found in cruciferous vegetables: broccoli, cauliflower, Brussels sprouts, and cabbage. They didn't find any in steak.

Or how about this headline that jumped off the page at me: oj fights breast cancer.[143] New research at the University of Western Ontario shows this to be so. And what component in the orange juice accomplishes this feat? Small molecules known as flavonoids, found in all citrus fruits.

Dr. Gladys Block, of the University of California at Berkeley, reviewed approximately 90 studies relating vitamin C intake and cancer. She indicated that, "There is overwhelming evidence of the protective effect of vitamin C and other antioxidants against cancer." Fruits and vegetables such as citrus fruits, tomatoes, green leafy vegetables, and potatoes are rich sources of vitamin C and other nutrients. Additionally, Dr. Block reviewed 170 studies from 17 nations and concluded that people everywhere who eat the most fruit and vegetables, compared with those who eat the least, slash their chances of developing cancer by about 50 percent![144] The evidence is so overwhelming that Dr. Block views fruits and vegetables as a powerful preventive that could substantially wipe out the scourge of cancer, just as cleaning up the water supply eliminated past epidemics such as cholera.

Dr. Peter Greenwald, director of the Division of Cancer Prevention and Control at the National Cancer Institute, Washington, D.C., says, "The more fruit and vegetables people eat, the less likely they are to get cancer, from colon and stomach cancer to breast and even lung cancer. For many cancers, persons with high fruit and vegetable intake have about half the risk of people with low intake."[145]

Dr. David Kritchevsky, in the journal *Cancer,* states that, "Breast cancer might be prevented if more women were to get sufficient amounts of Vitamin A, beta carotene and the other carotenoids."[146] Carotenoids are found in parsley, carrots, winter squash, sweet potatoes, yams, cantaloupe, apricots, spinach, kale, turnip greens, and citrus fruits.

Geoffrey R. Howe of the National Cancer Institute of Canada reviewed twelve case-controlled studies of diet and cancer and reported that fruits and vegetables provided a protective effect. Vitamin C showed the most consistent statistically significant inverse association with breast cancer risk in all women.[147]

In *Medical Tribune,* two studies indicated that nutrients, fiber, and antioxidants in fruits and vegetables protect women from cancer. One study found that of 310 women with breast cancer and 316 women without breast cancer, those without cancer ate more fruits and vegetables.[148]

Dr. Bruce N. Ames is a member of the National Academy of Sciences. He is a biochemist and molecular biologist at the University of California at Berkeley, where he is the director of the National Institute of Environmental Health Center. Dr. Ames is one of the two dozen most-often cited scientists in the world.[149] His colleagues refer to him as "one of the most innovative thinkers in the world of science."[150] Dr. Ames states that the antioxidant nutrients in fruits and vegetables "can suppress all stages of the cancer process," and that "diet is at least as important as smoking as a cause of cancer."[151]

A recent study on cancer prevention was conducted at the Memorial Sloan-Kettering Cancer Center in New York, and appeared in the *Journal of the National Cancer Institute* in October 1995. Dr. William R. Fair of Sloan-Kettering said, "What we found was astonishing to us."[152] And what was it that Dr. Fair found so astonishing? It is that human prostate cancer tumors grew only *half* as fast in mice eating diets that contained about 21 percent fat as those eating diets that contained about 40 percent fat.

Are you starting to see the picture here? Could there be any doubt in anyone's mind that it is at the very least a good idea to minimize intake of fat and maximize intake of plant foods? How much proof is enough?

Once again, here are a few comments from people involved in cancer research on one level or another.

Women on low fat diets have less breast cancer than women on high fat diets, and women on high fiber diets have less breast cancer than women on low fiber diets.[153]

—Dr. Lawrence Power,
author and syndicated food
and fitness columnist

If I were to blame anything for the modest increase in
breast cancer that is not related to early detection, I'd
point to dietary fat.[154]

> —Dr. Ernst Winder,
> President of the American Health
> Foundation

In terms of fat in the diet, there are several different
types of evidence—none of them completely conclusive,
but all of them pointing in the same direction—that link
a very low fat diet, really about half of what the average
American woman eats now, 20% of the total calories, to
a lower incidence of breast cancer.[155]

> —Cindy Pearson, Director, National
> Women's Health Network

As far as diet is concerned, while various investigators
have looked into the question of fat in relation to breast
cancer, none of them have examined the very much
more important questions that fat and fatty meat contain
high concentrations of pesticides, sex hormones, and
steroids, which are clearly known to induce cancer,
including cancer of the breast.[156]

> —Samuel Epstein, M.D.,
> Professor of Medicine, University of
> Chicago Medical Center

There is no such thing as a "Cancer Personality,"
although certain life-style choices—choosing to smoke
or eat a fatty diet, for instance—do make a difference.[157]

> —Jimmie Holland, M.D.,
> Memorial Sloan-Kettering Cancer
> Center

One study monitored more than 14,000 women for six years, focusing on their consumption of meat, fat, protein, and other animal products. Paolo Toniolo, of the New York Univer-sity Medical Center, who headed the study, said, "It seems that fre-quent meat consumers are at more of a risk for cancer. I don't know if it's fat or other elements of one's diet. But I know it's diet."[158]

And this final statement made on the nationally televised show "Nightline" by Dr. Timothy Johnson—truly the voice of common sense and reason:

You can probably lower your risk (of cancer) by cutting down on the fat in your diet. And even if we can't prove that either way, it makes sense to do it for all kinds of other reasons, so why not do it?[159]

Hear, hear. Why not, indeed?

I don't want to leave you with the idea that all cholesterol and all fat are harmful. The fact is, both are a requirement for life to continue. Cholesterol is not a harmful substance as such. It is used in all of the body's tissues. It occurs in the brain, spinal column, and skin. Cholesterol is part of the raw materi-als from which bile salts, sex and adrenal hormones, and vitamin D are made. It combines with proteins to enable fats to be carried to the cells. So important is cholesterol to life that the liver produces what it needs every single day. It's only the cholesterol taken into the body when we eat animal products that presents a danger.

Fats also must be viewed in the proper context. It may come as a surprise to you, but all foods contain fat. *All.* Even foods like watermelon, cucumbers, and apples. A certain amount of fat in the diet is an outright necessity. Vitamins A, D, E, and K cannot be utilized in the body except in the pres-ence of fat. They are "fat soluble," whereas vitamins such as B and C are "water soluble." Even if no fat is specifically eaten, the body can manufacture most of its required fatty acids from fruit and vegetable sugars. (A fatty acid is to fat what amino acids are to protein, the building blocks.) There are, however, two fatty acids that cannot be synthesized by the body and must be obtained from our diet. They are omega-6 (linoleic) and omega-3 (linolenic).

As it happens the omega-6 fatty acid is quite abundant in the typical western diet. It's in fruit, vegetables, legumes, whole grains, and vegetable oils. It's the omega-3 fatty acid that we do not consume nearly enough. The best sources of omega-3 include coldwater fish such as salmon, sardines, mackerel, herring, tuna, swordfish, and halibut, as well as soybeans, nuts (especially walnuts), flaxseeds and flaxseed oil, pumpkin seeds, hemp seeds, leafy green vegetables, and broccoli. I want you to bear in mind that exactly how omega-3 works in the body is not yet fully understood, which is why there is no established recommended daily intake. But it has been shown that people who regularly eat omega-3–rich fish have lower cholesterol levels and a lower incidence of cardiovascular disease by 40 percent or more.[160] It is also believed to be effective against psoriasis, arthritis, diabetes, migraines, and cancer. Evidently it also reduces LDL levels (bad cholesterol) while raising HDL (good cholesterol) levels.

Some people have started to take fish oil capsules to increase their omega-3 intake. But be forewarned: There are many potential problems associated with these supplements. Too much can bring on a stroke, and some actually contain cholesterol, thereby raising blood cholesterol levels. Also, it is well-known that fish oils are notorious for accumulating toxins, the very thing we are endeavoring not to do. The only established fact about fish oils is that they are a good source of omega-3.

Our goal then is not to eliminate fat; some fat is necessary for life. It is the *over*consumption of animal products that are extremely high in cholesterol and fat that poses the greatest threat to your health. At the end of the day, every day, determine where the bulk of your food intake came from, the animal kingdom or the plant kingdom. The evidence is in and is incontrovertible: your chances of living a long, pain-free, disease-free life, are absolutely increased when plant foods, not animal foods, predominate in your diet. This is notwithstanding the monstrous absurdities to be found in the high protein, low-carb, no fruit Death Diet.

THE CHINA HEALTH PROJECT

Over the years, there have been thousands of studies supporting what is now becoming common knowledge about the negative impact of animal products in the human diet. What makes a credible study? There are various criteria, including the length of the study, the number of people studied, the precision of the data collected, the means by which data are classified, the exactness with which the entire study is conducted, and to what extent each variable affects the overall outcome.

Because it is so difficult to conduct a study that is exemplary in all the above respects, for decades researchers have hoped for one study that linked diet to health that was so large-scale and definitive in every aspect it would be viewed by everyone as absolutely precise and unquestionably accurate. The days of hoping are over. Just such a study was inaugurated in 1983, and in mid-1990 the first seven years of its data were released. It is called the Cornell Oxford China Project on Nutrition, Health and Environment, known simply as the China Health Project (CHP).[161] In one of the many reviews of this extraordinary study, it is referred to as the "Grand Prix of Epidemiology."[162] In another article, it is called "The Champion Diet" and is hailed as "one of the most rigorous and conclusive studies in the history of health research."[163]

At my seminars, I always ask my audiences how many people have heard of the China Health Project. Even in audiences of more than a thousand people, only a smattering of hands go up. What an injustice! Considering its importance and potential benefit to people everywhere, this study should have been headlined on the front page of every newspaper in the world and been the leading story on every news program for at least a week, or for however long it took to be certain that every global citizen was aware of it.

If there is a true hero in the area of research linking diet to health, it is surely Dr. T. Colin Campbell, a nutritional bio-chemist at Cornell University, and mastermind and coordinator of the China Health Project. Dr. Campbell has been studying diet and health for more than a quarter of a century. He was instrumental in producing the National Academy of Sciences' landmark 1982 report, *Diet, Nutrition and Cancer,* which was the first "official" recommendation to reduce fat intake some 25 percent and which led to the guidelines adopted by the National Cancer Institute, the American Cancer Society, and the American Institute for Cancer Research. Although Dr. Campbell's innovative and groundbreaking research into the link between diet and health frequently met with opposition, his perseverance and commitment never wavered. Those traits brought him to the forefront of this area of research and made him one of the world's leading nutritional experts.

One of the factors that makes the China Health Project unique is the sheer scope of the study. Dr. Campbell, together with researchers from Oxford University and researchers commissioned by the Chinese government, observed 6,500 Chinese citizens for six years to obtain the widest possible range of data on death rates for more than fifty diseases, making the CHP the most complex study ever conducted of a single large population.

Undoubtedly the most striking aspect of the study and the element that has made it so reliable is the lifestyle of the study's Chinese subjects. Chinese people have two traits that helped make the research as exacting as it was. First, they generally do not move around. They are born, live, and die in the same locale. Second, their eating habits rarely vary. They eat essentially the same foods their entire lives with very little, if any, variation. Their diets are simple and basic, determined by the season. These factors allowed researchers to study a human laboratory on a very large scale for a very long time.

Perhaps you are familiar with the term "diseases of affluence." These include heart disease, cancer, diabetes, osteoporosis, and obesity. Throughout the world, whenever enough wealth allows people to move away from their basic needs, the prevalence of these diseases increases. In the United States, diseases of affluence are rampant. In China, they are either practically nonexistent or notably uncommon.

It is not a secret that the more affluent and industrialized a society, the more animal products and refined foods its people consume. Americans consume 16 million animals, 165 million eggs, 11 million pounds of fish, and 345 million pounds of dairy products every single day![164] The United States leads the world in diseases of affluence. In contrast, the Chinese primarily eat the cleansing foods: vegetables, grains and legumes, some fish, and no dairy. What is of inestimable importance is that they obtain 7 percent of their protein from animal products, while Americans obtain *70 percent* of their protein from animal products. Ten times as much!

The major reason Americans eat so much animal protein is that over the years they have been effectively conditioned to believe that protein every single day—indeed, every single meal—is absolutely essential for their health, and that animal products are the very best source of that protein. So, many people are running fat and cholesterol through their arteries, *every four hours.* It would be as though a car manufacturer were to somehow convince you through false advertising that you couldn't get a safe car unless you bought one of theirs. And the propaganda works so well that you're actually scared to buy a car from another source, even though you might be able to buy a vehicle as safe or safer than the one you are conditioned to buy.

The idea that it is difficult to obtain sufficient protein from the plant kingdom is an outright falsehood perpetuated by the industries that make money selling animal products and by their hired "experts." Millions of dollars have been spent over the years to condition you to automatically think of meat and other animal products whenever you think of protein. One of the most frequently asked questions of a vegetarian is, "Where do you get your protein?" As if by not eating animal products the nutrient can't be obtained. The conditioning has worked all too well.

The China Health Project rather soundly obliterates that particular profit-driven nutritional myth. In *Eat for Life: The Food & Nutrition Board's Guide to Reducing Your Risk of Chronic Disease,* published by the prestigious National Academy of Sciences, Dr. Paul R. Thomas writes, "There is nothing nutritionally unique about meat products that other foods cannot supply."[165] Dr. William E. Connor, author and head of the Division of Endocrinology, Metabolism and Nutrition at Oregon's Health Sciences University in Portland, sums it up well by saying, "The public has been sold on the idea that protein from animals is best and doesn't realize that plants contain high quality protein. Everything that grows has protein."[166] After all, isn't that where the animals we eat get theirs?

Heart disease in China declines to an almost negligible level when fat and cholesterol levels are low. The China Health Project shows that a low-fat and low-cholesterol diet protects not only against heart disease, but also against cancer of the colon. The more animal products eaten, the greater the risk to human health.

Obesity is a rarity in China. Although the Chinese consume 20 percent more calories than North Americans do, North Americans are 25 percent fatter! I have long maintained that calories are not a significant factor in whether you get fat or not. I was even attacked for saying so. The China Project and other data (see *T-Factor Diet* by Dr. Martin Katahn) certainly substantiate my point. After all, a calorie is nothing more than a measure of heat. Heat does not make you fat. Fat makes you fat. Unfortunately, it is being consistently shown that fat can also make you dead! Researchers show that as the obesity rate increases, so does the death rate.

Another area of great global concern, especially for women,

is osteoporosis, the loss of calcium from the bones until they become so porous and weak that a rib or hip can be broken merely by driving over a bump in the road. In the same way that we have been conditioned to think of meat whenever the word "protein" is mentioned, we have also been taught to believe that dairy products are the finest source of calcium, and the best means by which to prevent osteoporosis. That is precisely what the dairy industry, which makes billions of dollars selling dairy products, wants you to believe and once again it is patently untrue. It is a well established fact that the high protein content of meat and dairy products turns the blood acidic, which draws calcium out of the bones. This causes the body to lose or excrete more calcium than it takes in. The deficit must be made up from the body's calcium reserve, which is primarily the bones. Result—osteoporosis. This is not new information. It's been known since 1920 that protein from meat consumption causes a net loss of calcium.[167] Fortunately, protein from vegetable sources does not cause a negative calcium balance and, in fact, can actually have a protective effect against bone loss.[168]

Women who are eating dairy products to prevent osteo-porosis must pay attention to this well documented fact: The countries of the world that consume the greatest amount of dairy products have the highest incidence of osteoporosis! The countries that consume the lowest amount of dairy products have the lowest incidence of osteoporosis.[169] The United States is among the world's leading consumers of dairy products and has the highest incidence of osteoporosis, affecting between 15 and 20 million people and taking at least 20,000 lives a year as a result of hip fractures alone.[170]

The Chinese diet has changed since these studies were done, but at that time, according to Dr. Tierry Brun, an agricultural and nutritional scientist from the National Institute of Health and Medical Research in France, the Chinese consumed no cow's milk or dairy products, yet they had among the lowest rates of osteoporosis in the world.[171]

Dr. T. Colin Campbell pointed out that "dairy calcium is not needed to prevent osteoporosis. Most Chinese consume no dairy products and, instead, get all their calcium from vegetables. The Chinese data indicate that people need less calcium than we think and can get adequate amounts from vegetables."[172] As mentioned above, isn't that where the animals we eat get theirs!

For how many years have you been subjected to the aggressive propaganda by the dairy industry and their paid "experts" to frighten you, especially if you are a woman, into consuming dairy products lest you suffer the horror of osteoporosis? How much more sinister do those deceptive advertisements turn out to be now that it is becoming more obvious every day that protein and dairy products *contribute* to osteoporosis?

Yet another scare tactic employed by the animal products industry is its claim that red meat and other animal products are the best source of iron and that, without animal products, one risks developing anemia. The truth is that even in vegetarians and vegans, iron deficiency anemia is rare. In fact, studies reveal that they have iron levels as high or higher than those who eat an animal-based diet.[173] Moreover, vitamin C, which increases iron absorption from food, occurs in plant foods, not animal foods.[174]

The China Health Project sheds much-needed light on this subject as well. Those in the study "with the highest fiber intake also had the most iron rich blood."[175] You must understand that red meat, or any animal product for that matter, contains no fiber. The CHP also shows that "consumption of meat is not needed to prevent iron deficiency anemia. The average Chinese who shows no evidence of anemia consumes twice the iron Americans do, but the vast majority comes from the iron in plants."[176] Once again, isn't that where the animals we eat get theirs?

Another important finding was that the breast cancer death rate for American women is not double, triple, or even quadruple what it is for Chinese women, but a whopping five times the number of deaths. That is a 500 percent higher death rate.

Remember, Chinese women obtain 7 percent of their protein from animal products, while North American women obtain 70 percent of their protein from animal products. It is not time to sit around and wait for further evidence. It is time to take action and take the steps to protect yourself now!

As part of the National Institutes of Health's Women's Health Initiative, some 4,000 women will be tested to see if cutting dietary fat by half can lower breast cancer rates. They expect their results in the year 2006.[177] *You can't wait that long! The time is now!*

RESULTS OF THE CHINA HEALTH PROJECT

The results of this extraordinary study could not be clearer. The massive amount of industry-initiated, profit-driven propaganda that we have been inundated with over the years extolling the virtues of a diet laden with animal products has been instrumental in the toxification of your body and the deterioration of your health. The animal products industry has been well served. You haven't. The relationship is clear: The more animal products you eat, the more ill health ensues. Dr. Campbell reveals that:

> In those few regions in China where meat and dairy consumption has begun to increase—notably the heavily westernized cities—it has been closely followed by a higher incidence of cancer, heart disease and diabetes. Once these people start eating more animal products, that's when all the mischief starts.[178]

What has been demonstrated most clearly by the meticulously conducted China Health Project and what cannot be altered by the animal products industry's posturing and propaganda is that those who eat the least amount of animal products have the least risk of disease. Those who eat the most animal products have the highest rate of diseases of affluence. It is interesting to note that complex carbohydrates, which are only to be found in plant foods and never in animal foods, are the only food category not in some way linked to dread diseases.[179]

Today, the recommendations we are receiving from every quarter are to *decrease* our intake of food high in cholesterol and fat (animal products) and *increase* our consumption of foods high in fiber (fruit, vegetables, legumes, and whole grains). Remember that animal products are extremely high in cholesterol and fat, which clog you up, and are virtually devoid of fiber, which cleans you out! In other words, animal products could not be in more direct opposition to what researchers the world over are recommending we eat.

Having masterminded the China Health Project, having spent seven years in close contact with the accumulation and deciphering of its data, and having seen firsthand the result of this project, what does Dr. Campbell suggest we do to best prevent disease and preserve our health? As relates to diet, he recommends, "Change the diet so that 80% to 90% of protein comes from plant products, only 10% to 20% from animal products. Build meals around plant foods such as fruits, vegetables, grains and pasta. The idea is to use animal products to flavor and as an accompaniment, not as the main focus."[180]

As relates to exercise, Dr. Campbell recommends, "Exercise more. Chinese people are more physically active than people in the United States. They ride bicycles every day."[181] These are the basic guidelines of the program you will soon be following (see Part II).

Dr. Campbell sums up what he learned from the China Health Project as follows:

"We must come to realize that we are basically a vegetarian species. The study suggests that whether industrialized societies such as ours can cure themselves of their meat addiction, may ultimately be a greater factor in world health than all the doctors, health insurance policies, and drugs put together."[182]

Many of you are already cutting back your consumption of

animal products. Whether it's due to an "instinctive" knowledge that one should eat less meat and dairy, or the fact that more progressive physicians are now regularly encouraging it, or that news from the numerous studies supporting such a change is filtering down to the public, it is clear that people are consuming a less animal-based diet. How often do you hear others say, and how many of you can yourselves say, "I have definitely cut down on red meat and I'm eating more fish and chicken"? That is part of the trend, and that trend is validated and encouraged by a rapidly growing number of authorities both outside and inside the medical community.

If you have not yet joined this trend because you feel the issue is not quite settled or that the "experts" are still at odds, your time has arrived. It would be a formidable challenge to find anyone other than those making money from their sale who does not agree that reducing animal products in the diet is a wise decision. Take the American Dietetic Association. In its position paper on vegetarianism, the organization makes it clear that even if you wanted to become a strict vegetarian, you could do so confidently by eating from a wide range of nonanimal foods.[183] If the journey all the way to vegetarianism is safe, obviously only cutting back would pose no problem.

Comments on vegetarianism from places where not even ten years ago you would never have expected to hear them are beginning to surface. Where do you think the following statement comes from?

> Although we think we are one, and we act as if we are one, human beings are not natural carnivores. When we kill animals to eat them, they wind up killing us because their flesh was never intended for human beings who are natural herbivores.[184]

Are these the words of someone clinging to the "sixties"? Are they the words of the head of one of the many animal rights groups in America? Wrong on both counts. They are the words of Dr. William C. Roberts, professor of clinical medicine at Georgetown University and chief cardiology pathologist for the National Institutes of Health. He also happens to be the editor-in-chief of the *American Journal of Cardiology,* a conservative, mainstream medical journal. The above statement appeared in an editorial in that journal and it should prompt us to wonder how we could have ever been so misled.

Sometimes change is difficult. It certainly is when the change runs counter to what we have been used to doing for years, *decades,* but the change of reducing the overall amount of animal products in your diet can have only one long-term effect: a longer, healthier, disease-free life. That is why one of the principles of CARE deals with how to accomplish this in the most effective and convenient way possible.

To be perfectly clear on the subject, I am not saying you have to become a vegetarian, which is clearly not for everyone. What I am saying is that many people are overeating on animal products and it would be wise to cut back. The second principle in the CARE program will assist you in that effort.

As discussed in Chapter Five, the lymph system plays an invaluable role in the prevention of all disease. That being so, make the following two things priorities: First, strive to do whatever you can to reduce the burden on your lymph system; and second, strive to do whatever you can to optimize the lymph system's functioning.

As regards the first point, one of the major, basic functions of the lymph system is to absorb fats from the digestive tract.[185] The more fat you eat, the harder your lymph system has to work, the more clogged it becomes, and the less energy it has for the cleansing and removal of wastes. So the less it has to remove, the better.

As regards the second point, there is something you can do to directly assist and support your lymph system's optimum operation and effectiveness. It is an ingredient that is indispensable to a healthy lifestyle and imperative for the activities of the lymph system. That ingredient is, of course, exercise.

NINE

Exercise

Hold it! Before you pass up this chapter with something like, "Yeah, yeah, I should exercise. I know. I'll read this later," just read a little of it now, please. Later has a funny way of turning into never, and I promise not to beat you over the head with a celebrity workout tape. I know darn good and well that if you're not exercising, one more admonishment that you'd better start is probably not going to get you out huffing and puffing.

So what I'd like to do is tell you something about exercising that you are probably not aware of and offer you such a simple, effective means of exercising that you just couldn't stay sedentary. Besides, I could hardly write a book on health care and not include exercise. The relationship between a healthy life and regular exercise is irrefutable. Consider the fact, for example, that exercisers have an all-cause mortality rate that is less than one-third that of nonexercisers.[186] Moreover, some form of regular physical activity, even if it's a very mild form of activity, is crucial for vibrant health. Here's why: Exercise helps your lymph system function at an optimal level.

Unlike the cardiovascular system, which has at its center the heart acting as a pump to keep the flow of blood going, the lymph system has no such pump. But lymph fluid must constantly be flowing throughout the body, in the same way that blood must constantly be flowing throughout the body. Remember, there is three times more lymph fluid in your body than blood. What is it that does for the lymph system what the heart does for the cardiovascular system? Physical activity. *Exercise!*[187] The flow of lymph through the body is also helped by the muscles in the walls of lymph vessels and by respiration (breathing in and out), but the important contribution of exercise cannot be overstated. This information should put the need for regular physical activity in a whole new light.

Most people, whether they exercise or not, are aware of the value of exercise in supporting a healthy lifestyle. One of the most important and convincing studies supporting this fact and reported in the *Journal of the American Medical Association* by a group of highly respected researchers, including exercise guru Dr. Kenneth H. Cooper, studied the exercise habits of more than 13,000 men and women for more than eight years. Their physical fitness was measured by a treadmill exercise task. The study showed that the all-causes death rate of the least fit men was three times that of the fittest men; with women, this rate was five times higher. The data showed that an unfit man could reduce his risk of death from all diseases by nearly 37 percent by becoming fit, and an unfit woman could reduce her risk by about 48 percent![188] Those are figures that are hard to ignore.

Yet, with this and so many other studies proving the life-extending benefits of exercise, at last count, less than 10 percent of the nation's adults exercise vigorously at least three times a week.[189] Why? It's not simply a communication problem, to be sure. Nonexercisers know they need to exercise.

How often have you heard, or even said yourself, "I know I

need to exercise, but . . ." Let's face it, there are probably many reasons, physical, emotional, and psychological, why people don't exercise. It's not necessary to delve into all the reasons. What is important is to somehow get those people who are the most sedentary sufficiently motivated to do at least something.

If you are already doing some form of exercise, no matter how little or how much, that's fine. What I wish to accomplish here is to get those of you doing practically nothing up and moving. You see, it doesn't take that much. There's no reason to feel intimidated. You don't have to join a gym or take aerobics classes. Really, I'm not suggesting you become a world-class athlete. But I will tell you this, and I won't soften what I'm about to say. Are you serious about doing what you can to live a vibrantly healthy life free of the pain, anguish, and suffering that disease can cause? If your answer is yes, and you are serious, and I mean *really* serious, then you must do everything you can to keep your lymph system operating at its highest possible efficiency, and some form of regular physical exercise is a major contributing factor in that effort. Period! There's no way around it. Exercise is the key.

WALKING

There is one vigorous, physical activity that can bring you all the benefits afforded by exercise, can be done practically anywhere at any time, by nearly anyone, regardless of physical condition, doesn't require elaborate facilities or equipment, and is convenient and easy. It is walking!

Walking produces results in short-term training and in long-term health benefits equal to any other aerobic exercise—including jogging![190] When you jog, you land with 3 or 4 times your body weight. When you walk, you always have one foot on the ground and, therefore, land with only 1 to 1½ times your body weight. As joggers age, they increasingly experience knee, ankle, and back injuries. Walking is far easier on the joints and bones.

All around the world, walking has been a popular and recognized means of keeping fit. At the turn of the twentieth century, one of the most grueling competitive events in the United States was the "six day race." Edward Payson Weston was the most popular walking champion of the day. He would regularly cover more than 400 miles in those competitions and his fans lined the route and cheered him on all the way. In 1904, at age seventy-one, he walked across the United States from San Francisco to New York in 104 days, walking on average over 40 miles a day. Mr. Weston passed away at age ninty-one, leaving the legacy of the "evening constitutional" as a part of the American way of life.[191]

At that same time Theodore Roosevelt was considered to be one of the fittest presidents ever. Vigorous exercise helped him overcome serious childhood health problems, and he exercised regularly and encouraged exercise throughout his life. In 1909, at the end of his presidency, he demonstrated his physical fitness by walking 50 miles in three days.[192]

At the beginning of the twentieth century, heart attacks became increasingly prevalent. This devastating health problem was so thoroughly misunderstood that doctors actually thought physical activity made the heart wear out and, astonishingly, discouraged heart attack victims from physical activity.[193] Those afflicted were told to rest and remain inactive, the very worst possible advice. The heart, which is a muscle, requires regular exercise to keep it strong and make it stronger. But more than thirty years would pass before this understanding would take hold.

In 1924, Dr. Paul Dudley White founded the American Heart Association and is considered to be the "father of American cardiology." He stunned his colleagues by saying that not only was walking *not* dangerous, it was, in fact, absolutely beneficial and people should be encouraged to take daily walks. This statement was made at a time when cardiology patients were forced to lie flat on their backs with as little movement as possible for six weeks! Doctors theorized that it would take that long for the heart to heal.

This bedrest theory was disputed by Dr. White because he noticed too many complications from such prolonged inactivity. After all, the human body is beautifully designed for activity and does not deal well with six weeks of forced inactivity. Another three decades would pass before changes were actually made in medical treatment for heart attack patients. Dr. White, of course, was already encouraging his patients to get out of bed and start a program of walking.

Probably the most well-known studies on risk factors involved in heart disease are the Framingham studies started in the 1950s in Framingham, Massachusetts. There, researchers studied approximately 10,000 people for more than thirty years and amassed a wealth of information that began to reveal the important role of activity in preventing heart disease. Many more studies have been subsequently conducted and today the inescapable fact is that regular physical activity is needed to ensure good health and prevent heart disease, the country's Number 1 killer. After all, as one study conducted by the Centers for Disease Control revealed, people who do not exercise have twice the risk of developing heart disease as those who do.[194]

Walking is the ideal aerobic exercise, one that oxygenates the blood which, in turn, supplies oxygen to all cells of the body. The Number 1 prerequisite of life is air. Weeks can go by without food, days without water, but only a few minutes without air before you die. The literal meaning of the word "aerobic" is "in the presence of air." The heart, lungs, and blood vessels work in harmony to carry this life-giving oxygen to every part of the body.

When you walk, you use your body's large muscles, which allow the entire aerobic mechanism of your body to work harder than when you are at rest. If this exercise is done consistently, over time, the system becomes stronger and ever more efficient and capable of performing the functions it was designed to perform. Over a lifetime, walking is the best possible means of reducing the risk of cardiovascular disease. Add to that the fact that walking will stimulate the activity of your lymph system, and you have a real winner in this exercise.

Truly exciting and encouraging are the recent studies showing that even the most moderate, unstructured walking program will reap substantial benefits. Of course, common sense should tell you that the more you do, the more vigorously, the more benefit you will enjoy. But the good news, the great news, is that even low levels of activity are beneficial. For example, in one of the first clinical studies of its kind, as reported in the *Journal of the American Medical Association,* it was shown that regular hour-long strolls will reduce a woman's risk of heart disease.[195] Mile for mile, walking is actually the best fat burner.[196] Walking four miles burns more fat than running the same distance in less time![197] An editorial in the same journal points out that a brisk twenty-minute walk three times a week produces many benefits.[198] Dr. James Gavin, author of *The Exercise Habit,* maintains that, "Ten minutes of extra activity per day can reduce an individual's risk of heart disease by 80%."[199]

Considering the subject of this book, and this chapter, imagine my excitement when I was looking through the *New York Times* one morning and the following headline jumped off the page: STUDY LINKS EXERCISE TO DROP IN BREAST CANCER. The results of the study were published in the *Journal of the National Cancer Institute* and stated, "A thorough new study has found that moderate but regular physical activity can reduce a woman's risk of developing premenopausal breast cancer by as much as 60%.[200] Sixty percent! In a discussion of the study on the "NBC Network News," it was stated that "the researchers are saying that exercise is the most important step a woman can take to reduce her risk of breast cancer."[201]

Three years later there was a report in the *New England Journal of Medicine* about another major study that followed

25,000 women for fourteen years. The study concluded: "Compared with sedentary women, those who exercised at least four hours a week had a 37% lower risk of developing breast cancer, and the more women exercised, the less likely they were to develop the disease." The executive director of the Center for Cancer Prevention at Harvard University said, "This is a new, quite powerful piece of eveidence."[202] There simply is no longer any reason not to do *some* walking.

GET WALKING

I suggest a program of walking that is very unstructured, quite easy, and will satisfy your body's need for exercise and support your efforts to achieve vibrant health. This is not a contest—you are not being graded on your effort, and no one will be "looking over your shoulder" to check up on you. This is your chance to do what you know in your heart is so important, without pressure and without guilt. You do as much or as little as you choose for your own comfort. Anything helps!

All that is required is an agreement with yourself that you *will* do something. Your goal should be to build up to a 30- to 45-minute easy walk three or four times a week, *at your own pace.* That's it! Perhaps in the beginning you will find it easier if you make your walks functional. Turn them into an errand to pick up some lightweight odds and ends at the store or to mail a letter. Sometimes getting used to walking is easier if you have a purpose and destination.

There are other ways to integrate walking into your lifestyle. On occasion, you can leave early enough for work in the morning to park a mile or so from your place of employment and walk the rest of the way. That walk, coupled with the return walk at the end of the day, will not only fulfill your daily exercise requirement but will also allow you to feel invigorated when you arrive at work and perked up when you return home. Or you can incorporate a walk into your lunch routine, especially during the winter, when extreme cold in the morning and darkness after work might keep you indoors.

In addition, whenever you can, walk upstairs instead of taking an elevator. Stair-climbing is an excellent workout that also helps keep your legs in good shape, and you will benefit from even brief stair-climbing efforts. Drive to a park for the sole purpose of taking a walk in fresh air and pleasant surroundings. Any way or at any time that you can walk, no matter how much or how little, do it! It all adds up physically, and psychologically the feeling of accomplishment will be immeasurably worthwhile.

WALKING HINTS

To optimize your results, consider the following hints to make your walking experience the most enjoyable and productive it can possibly be:

1. At the top of the list, and possibly the most important factor for successful walking, is wearing the proper footwear. Contrary to what many people believe, walking is not merely running at a slower speed. The motion of walking is very different from that of running. The transfer of weight is not at all the same. It's a much slower rolling motion versus landing on your heel quickly, with more weight. Running shoes need to be softer; walking shoes need to be firmer. Just as running, tennis, soccer, and other sports require specifically designed shoes, so does walking. Take your walking seriously, and please buy the proper shoes! Cutting corners will be a big mistake. This is very important! Purchase a good pair, of which there are many brands, and they will pay for themselves many times over in comfort, enjoyment, and benefits.

I have found walking shoes made by ASICS to be the best. Although they are relatively new to the walking market, ASICS' shoes are the most innovative. Not only are these shoes particularly comfortable, they also have an exclusive, patented gel system in the soles and heels that disburses the vertical impact into a horizontal plane, absorbs shock, and dissipates vibration.

What really sold me on the uniqueness and efficacy of ASICS products was the experience of the great basketball hall-of-famer Rick Barry. Between his playing days and several operations on his knees, Rick was left with absolutely no cartilage in his knees, just bone against bone. He is very athletic; he plays basketball and tennis, and enjoys jogging. Due to the absence of cartilage in his knees, however, he could only engage in his favorite activities for very short periods of time and even that caused him considerable pain, requiring rest and ice packs. He told me that he had resigned himself to the fact that he was not going to be able to be as physically active as he would like. But then along came the ASICS gel sneakers and Rick can now play for hours without discomfort or need for ice packs. No pain. No damage. Amazing, and in Rick Barry's words, "a real miracle" for him.

2. When it's warm out, walk either in the early morning or late afternoon. Walking in the heat of the day is not a good idea because you not only absorb the heat directly from the sun, but also from the pavement. It's interesting to note that when exercise is performed in the morning, 75 percent of participants stick with it, versus 25 percent who drop it when exercise is scheduled for any other time of day.[203]

3. Don't push it. Take it easy at first. Start slowly and build up strength, especially if you have not been exercising regularly. Perhaps the first week or two, or the first month, you may not even go for 30 minutes or only walk twice a week. You don't have to prove anything to anyone. Remember, less than 10 percent of the nation's adults exercise vigorously three times a week!

The mere fact that you're doing it at all puts you in a very elite group, and you are to be commended. Your muscles are there to be used. It will not take long before they accustom themselves to the new activity and normalize. Yes, you may feel sore muscles at first, but this is a "good" soreness. You are using muscles that have been deprived of activity and are being "broken in," so to speak. Warm baths do wonders to alleviate initial strain.

4. If it is windy out, start your walk with the wind in your face and return with it at your back. This prevents your getting a chill as a result of the perspiration you've worked up.

5. Swing your arms. This helps circulate the blood and strengthen the heart. Ever notice how long music conductors live? When I hear of a music conductor passing away, he's usually in his eighties or nineties. Music conductors spend their lives swinging their arms, and heart disease is rare among them. Leonard Bernstein died in his sixties, unfortunately, but this was due to his addiction to cigarettes.

6. It is best if there is no food in your stomach when you are exercising. Digesting demands energy and detracts from your ability to exercise well. The exception is fruit, which requires very little energy to digest.

7. Dehydration can be a real problem in any form of exercise. You must drink water to replenish yourself. Your body is approximately 70 percent water, and as a normal course of events, you lose about 2 to 2½ quarts a day. That can go to 4 quarts if you exercise. Drink water, not soft drinks, Gatorade, or any of the other fluids that contain chemical substances that undermine health. Drink a glass of water before you walk and after you finish your walk. Drink more if you feel the need. It is better to take in a little more than you need than not to take in enough.

(For more information on the proper hydration of your body

and a beneficial water science that I am excited about, call 877-335-1509 or view the Web page: www.fitforlifetime.com/links.php.)

8. Stretching is an excellent habit to practice while walking or after your walk. Stretching can relieve stiffness, increase the range of motion of your muscles, and prevent injuries. Stretching should be performed only *after* your muscles have warmed up and should never go to the point of causing pain. Stretching can itself be of enormous benefit, and there are dozens of stretches. Here are three to try:

- Stretch your hamstrings on the back of your legs by bending over and touching your toes. If you can't touch your toes, just go as far as you can. Hold it for 15 to 20 seconds and come back up. Never bounce when you stretch.

  As far as you can go is fine. By doing this stretch regularly, you will be amazed at how soon you will be able to touch your toes with ease.
- Stretch your thighs by holding on to something for support with your left hand while, with your right hand, you pull your right foot up behind you toward your lower back. Then reverse.
- Stretch your calves by standing on the edge of a stair with only the front half of your foot on the stair, then sink your weight down on your heel.

Each of these three stretches can be repeated. You can't stretch too much, so do as much as you like.

One of the most attractive aspects of walking is the convenience of it. You can walk anywhere—on the street, around your house, near your office, in the woods or a park, or on country trails. No matter where you are, with no more than a good pair of walking shoes, you're always able to take advantage of this life-extending practice. What if you feel it is too hot or too cold to walk? Most malls open their doors quite early, hours before the stores are open. The temperature is always just right. The walking surface is flat and smooth, and malls are well lit and safe. It's almost as if they were designed for walking.

BENEFITS OF WALKING

Any way you look at it, walking is an enormously positive activity and can influence your life in many positive ways. The list of benefits you can reap from walking is definitely impressive. Consider:

1. It helps increase the strength and efficiency of your heart and muscles.[204]
2. A recent study indicates that walking lowers cholesterol.[205]
3. Walking, like other exercises, increases both energy level and stamina. Overall strength, flexibility, and balance are also improved.[206]
4. Walking actually increases bone mass.[207] Bones, like muscles, become stronger with regular exercise. It has been well established that the risk of osteoporosis is lowered with regular exercise.
5. Together with a healthy diet, walking can be instrumental in helping you lose weight. A 45-minute walk every other day for a year can burn 18 pounds of fat.[208]
6. According to Dr. James Rippe, walking reduces hypertension (high blood pressure) and aids diabetics.[209]
7. Walking, like other exercise, promotes better sleep.[210]
8. One study at a medical center in Salt Lake City showed that mild exercise such as walking after eating moved food through the stomach more quickly, helping to relieve minor indigestion.[211]

9. A study at Appalachian State University showed that women who walked 45 minutes a day recovered twice as fast from colds as women who did not exercise.[212]

10. According to the *Berkeley Wellness Letter,* walking is the perfect exercise for promoting a healthy back.[213]

11. Walking relieves stress. Researchers at the Center for Health and Fitness at the University of Massachusetts found that people who took a brisk 40-minute walk experienced a 14 percent average drop in anxiety levels. Walks are part of the therapy at the Betty Ford Center for Drug and Alcohol Rehabilitation.[214]

12. A study at the Exercise, Physiology and Human Performance Laboratory at the University of California at San Diego showed that healthy men ages thirty-five to sixty-five who started a regular exercise program hugged and kissed their wives more often and had more sexual intercourse and more orgasms than those who did not exercise.[215]

13. A growth hormone administered to people over the age of sixty reduces fat, increases bone mass, improves skin condition, and reverses many other apparent symptoms of aging. The artificial hormone is very expensive and has serious side effects, but walking as little as 20 minutes a day has been shown to stimulate this growth hormone production.[216]

14. Walking lowers blood pressure.[217]

15. Walking reduces the risk of colon cancer.[218]

16. Walking boosts the defense system.[219]

17. Walking stimulates the lymph system which, as you have learned, is essential in the prevention of disease.

One of the greatest rewards from a program of regular exercise such as walking is the mental and emotional lift it provides that spills over into the other areas of your life.

We all know the importance of exercise, and when we don't do any, not only do we suffer physiologically, we also suffer psychologically. Somewhere inside, we berate ourselves for not doing the right thing. That all changes when you start to walk. Instead of having a negative feeling every time you are reminded that you don't exercise sufficiently, you feel a surge of pride that you do. Your level of self-esteem grows steadily and a positive message resounds through you instead of a negative one. You start to exude happiness and healthfulness because you truly *are* happier and healthier. On every possible level, you are improving your health. The richest person in the world can't buy this feeling of well-being for any amount of money because its value transcends money. You can have this feeling starting right now for the price of a pair of shoes. Make the effort. You're worth it!

With walking or any other form of exercise, consistency is the key. Do it at a pace that suits you and doesn't put pressure on you. Don't let it be something that hangs over you as a kind of onerous responsibility. If you start slowly and engage in it moderately, walking will gradually become as normal and natural a part of your life as putting on clothes in the morning. You'll look forward to it. You'll miss it if you don't do it. Discover walking. Make it a part of your life, and you will never regret it.

OTHER EXERCISE

There are two other noteworthy ways in which you can assist the stimulation of your lymph system. The first is a technique called lymphatic drainage massage. Seek out a qualified massage therapist familiar with this technique. There are several areas of the body, on the legs, arms, torso, and neck that can be massaged to directly assist the lymph system in its effort to cleanse the body.

The second approach is rebounding, discussed in great detail in *Fit for Life II*. Rebounders, or "minitrampolines" as they are commonly called, can help you prevent disease, that's the greatest deal on earth. These Rebounders can be found on the Web site www.vpnutrition.com.

Rebounding is extremely easy. All it calls for is a slight up-and-down bounce, which subjects the body to a change in velocity and direction twice with each jump. At the bottom of the bounce, all the one-way valves of the lymph system are closed because of the pressure above them. At the top of the bounce, the valves are open, allowing the lymph to flow up as the body starts down. Every valve opens at the same time, allowing and stimulating the flow of lymph.[220] As little as five or six minutes a day can be of immeasurable value. I believe that rebounding is a superior way to stimulate lymph circulation and drainage. Unlike many other exercises, it is gentle and highly effective.

Anything you can do to assist your lymph system should be done. A little effort goes a long way.

Start now! Your body will thank you with renewed, good health.

Part II

The CARE Program

TEN

An Introduction to CARE

No matter how great-sounding a program for disease prevention is, no matter how convincing the argument to follow it is, no matter how promising the results will be if it is followed, if there is not a way to easily implement it and see results, all the swell-sounding promises are for naught. For decades, there have been numerous admonitions telling us over and over again *what* we have to do, and *why,* to experience the highest level of health. And although knowing what and why is of extreme importance, both are unhelpful, if not useless, unless accompanied by the *how* that will bring about the desired results.

The CARE program is the new path to vibrant health! At the heart of this approach are three principles which, if implemented regularly, will quickly prove their worthiness. Your health will change for the better and the evidence of this bold statement will make itself apparent in no uncertain terms. You will *feel* better, you will *look* better, and your lymph system will be clean and operating at a highly efficient level.

Bear in mind, however, that there are no magic formulas, although sometimes when the body is cleansed of wastes and toxins, the positive results do appear to be miraculous. But your body automatically brings about these "miracles" when you make the changes to facilitate them. As I said earlier, for change to occur, changes must be made. It's like the old saying: "If there is no change, then there is no change." We are talking about simple logic here. If you want your health to be different from what it has been, then there must be some changes made to make that a reality.

More often than not, I have found that people wanting change in their lives put far too much pressure on themselves, especially when the change calls for dietary modifications. For some reason, people put themselves in an "all-or-nothing" mode, diving into new behaviors with great resolve, restricting themselves too severely, and burning themselves out in a few weeks, quickly reverting to old habits that weren't working. The only thing different in their lives is some new guilt to deal with from not succeeding in this latest fling with health.

Some of you may conform to the above scenario when you start the three principles that are set out on the following pages. So before going any further, let me try to prevent as many of you as possible from falling into this trap: These principles are guidelines to help you, not edicts to hinder you. They are tools to assist you, not rules to enslave you.

Your effort to improve your health and prevent becoming sick needn't be a stress-filled journey. It can be a joyous one. This is not a race! The prize does not go to the one who gets there first. The prize goes to all who join the race! That is because the prize is the journey itself! It's not how fast you travel, it's that you even make the trip at all. You have time. More time than you need. You see, even if you make use of the three CARE principles in a very conservative way until you are comfortable with them and they become an integral part of your lifestyle, you will have changed your direction, and in so doing, disease will become less and less of a possibility in your life. Rather than stagnating or becoming a little unhealthier every day, allowing the disease process to progress, you will, with each passing day, know what it means to become a little healthier. Direction is everything. Speed is nothing.

Imagine you and your family pulling through the entrance gate at Yellowstone National Park. You could spend a week taking in the beauty of this awe-inspiring national treasure and still not see it all. Or you could race through it in half a day as though you were being chased by hungry bears. In either case, you could boast to your friends, "Yeah, we did Yellowstone." But which trip did you do? Which trip do you think would be most uplifting? The one in which you leisurely drink in the natural beauty that feeds your spirit and soul, or the one in which you screech through at breakneck speed throwing yourself and everyone with you into a panic of apprehension?

The principles I am about to share with you should not be viewed as a forced march, but rather as a light along your path. When it is convenient and comfortable to use them, do so. When it is not, don't. Know that to whatever degree you use these principles, however often you choose to implement them, that will be right for you, and they will serve you exactly as well as they will serve those who embrace them to a fuller or lesser degree than you. It's always better to do a little less at first and then do more as you start to see results than to try to do too much and have to cut back and feel as though you failed.

One thing you can count on if you use the three CARE principles: they will work! I have seen them do so for so many people for so many years. I'm one of them. So ready is your body, so well equipped and capable is it to acquire and maintain a consistent level of vibrant health when given the opportunity, that even with the most moderate adherence to these principles, you will start to experience the benefits that they can so effectively bring about.

THE HEALING POWER OF THE BODY

Throughout the book I have praised the nearly unfathomable magnificence and intelligence of the human body. I wish to return to this for just a moment before presenting the CARE principles. Earlier, I made the point that all of the endless activities of the body are sourced and monitored by the brain. It's amazing when you think about the fact that all the incredible advances made by the human species, from electricity to air travel, from automobiles to computers, all had their beginnings in the brain, and we only use about 10 to 15 percent of our brain. Wow! So, what is the remaining 85 to 90 percent of this spectacular gem of creation doing? You can be sure it's not merely there to take up space in our skulls.

The body's—the brain's—Number 1 priority at any and every given moment, is self-preservation. If the part of the brain used to figure out how to go to the moon at 17,000 miles per hour, play hopscotch, and come back is so small, can you even begin to imagine the power working for your well-being in the vast majority of your brain? Awesome! Your body will *never* give up on you. All you have to do is not stand in its way. In other words, all you have to do to benefit from its unparalleled power is support its natural inclination to seek out and maintain its highest level of health possible. The three principles of CARE, which are the subject of the next three chapters, provide that support.

Naturally, you want some kind of proof that these principles will indeed do what I claim. I could tell you about plenty of people who use the three CARE principles and have not gotten sick, but someone could easily say, "Well, how do you know it was the three principles that prevented it? Maybe it was because they liked to garden, or because they took vitamins, or because of any number of other activities they participated in." So, about the only proof I can offer is how the principles fare in either stopping, reversing, or banishing cancer once it has taken hold.

CASE STUDY

Over the years I have received hundreds of thousands of letters from people who have made truly remarkable recoveries in their health. I want to share with you a most extraordinary story that clearly demonstrates the indomitable spirit of one woman and the unparalleled healing ability of the human body. Her name is Anne Frahm. She wrote a book about her experiences. Here is her story.

Anne Frahm is a forty-six-year-old wife and mother of two. In her mid-thirties she started to experience an excruciating, unrelenting pain between her shoulder blades. X rays showed "hot spots" on the bones of her shoulder, which her doctor diagnosed as bursitis. The doctor also told her that her condition was being complicated by a kidney infection.

She was given cortisone shots, and was told to apply daily ice packs to her shoulder. She was also given heavy doses of antibiotics both orally and intravenously for the kidney infection. All that happened was that the pain became progressively worse. In fact, it became so bad that she could not roll over in bed or even hug her own children without experiencing unbearable pain.

This situation went on for seven months, at which time she went to a hospital emergency room to seek another doctor's opinion. This doctor conferred with Ms. Frahm's family doctor and they wondered if all this pain wasn't really just in her head. She was given a shot of muscle relaxant and a prescription for Valium, and sent home.

Still in pain, she demanded more definitive answers of her doctor. She was sent for a CAT scan. A young doctor came into her room with the results and told her she had advanced breast cancer to such a degree that she had to have a mastectomy the very next day! When she asked how bad it was, the doctor answered, "I'm not going to pull any punches; most people who have cancer so advanced die within two years."

It wasn't only hearing that she had breast cancer that so shocked her, it was also the fact that several months before the pain even began she had found a small lump in her breast during a self-examination. Since her grandmother had died of breast cancer and her mother had had both breasts removed because of ongoing, troubling cysts in her breasts, Anne had wasted no time in getting a mammogram. She was told that there were indeed two tiny lumps but they were benign, non-cancerous. An additional ultrasound test also confirmed that they were benign. The doctor said, "Nope, no cancer here."

Not only were they cancerous, but the cancer had spread and tumors were found covering her skull, shoulder, ribs, pelvis, and up and down her spine.

Her breast was removed along with a tumor that was beneath it, the size of her entire breast. For the next year and a half her body was subjected to varied treatments including high doses of chemotherapy and radiation. She went bald, developed severe pneumonia, and her skin from head to toe broke out into itchy, red splotches.

After all of her pain and suffering from the cancer, the chemo-therapy, and the radiation, she was told that the cancer was steadily progressing and that her situation was becoming ever worse. She was told that her last possible hope was a bone marrow transplant. I don't even want to begin to tell you what a horrendous experience such a procedure is. Suffice it to say that it is something you never want to experience.

A couple of months after the bone marrow transplant, monitoring of her white blood cell count indicated that there was still a lot of cancer in her marrow. Further chemotherapy was out of the question, as it would have killed her outright.

When she inquired about a new experimental drug being tested on some patients to stimulate the growth of white blood cells, she was given the most stunning, mind-numbing response imaginable: Since there was only a limited amount of the drug available, it had to be held in reserve for patients with a more favorable chance of survival. Sorry! With sadness and regret, she was sent home to die.

It is impossible to read Anne's account of her husband, her children, and herself huddled together, mourning her impending death, without weeping.

But Anne Frahm did not know the meaning of the words "give up." They weren't in her vocabulary. She loved her family and her life and was not ready to leave. Her last-ditch effort was to turn to a nutritionist for help. She was counseled, given books to read, put on a very strict, detoxifying diet, and never lost her positive attitude. She knew she was going to win. A mere five weeks later, in the most remarkable instance of self-healing I have ever encountered, not even the slightest trace of cancer could be found in her body. It was gone! Her doctor, noticeably flabbergasted, said, "When you returned from the trans-plant with cancer in your marrow, I honestly thought you were doomed!"

As word of Anne's miraculous recovery spread and doctors and laypeople alike kept contacting her to hear her story, she decided to put it all down in a book. That book is called *A Cancer Battle Plan,* and it was published in 1993.

Before I heard of either Anne or her book, she wrote me a letter and sent me a picture of herself. Looking at her smiling face and her full head of lush, black hair filled me with joy, as did her letter, which read:

Dear Harvey,

Thank you! Thank you! Thank you! You have helped save the life of this 46-year-old wife and mother—me! Ten years ago I was dying of cancer. After 1½ years of chemo-therapy, radiation, surgery, and even a bone marrow transplant, nothing worked and I was sent home to die. Instead, I consulted a nutritionist. FIVE WEEKS later at my next checkup, tests revealed NO TRACE of cancer in my body!! I've been cancer free and HEALTHY for ten years!

One of the first books my nutritionist recommended was *Fit for Life*. The simple, commonsense approach you use helped me and my husband form a basis of understanding that helped me overcome cancer. THANK YOU for standing up in the face of overwhelming opposition to tell the truth!!

Your greatest fan,
Anne Frahm

In order to overcome this severely advanced cancer, Anne detoxified her body through dietary regimentation (Principle 1 in the CARE program); entirely removed animal products from her diet (variation of Principle 2); and filled her mind with positiveness and prayer (Principle 3). The implications of this should be blindingly obvious to anyone interested in preventing cells from being driven crazy. If this woman, who was brought to death's door with no hope of survival, was able to use information similar to the information contained in this book to reverse and banish the cancer from her body, do you fully realize the power and ability you have to prevent cells from ever being driven crazy in the first place? I hope you do. I sincerely hope you see the control over your health the concepts in this book give you. If cancer can be reversed, it can be prevented. You *can* prevent disease! You *can* live in vibrant health!

Because this is a book primarily about prevention, many people have asked me whether or not existing illnesses they are dealing with can be cured by following the recommendations in the CARE program. My immediate inclination is to blurt out a resounding *yes!* By all means, yes! But I can't do that and I'd like to tell you why. There are laws that can deal very harshly with those who make statements about what can be expected by following a certain health regimen if the person making the statements is not a medical doctor. The fact is, I, and anyone else in the health movement not in possession of a medical degree, must be exceedingly careful how we impart what we have learned, so as not to be accused of practicing medicine without a license. This is irrespective of the validity of what is being suggested. The reason I reprinted Ms. Frahm's letter relating how she reversed such advanced cancer is because there are no laws preventing someone from discussing their own personal experiences. So bear in mind what I'm about to impart has been very, *very* carefully thought out so that I don't get myself in trouble.

You've heard it before: The only things guaranteed in life are taxes and death. Everything else is open for discussion. The truth is, whether a medical doctor or not, no one can make any guarantees about what will or will not, or what can or can not happen when it comes to the health and healing of the human body. There are simply far too many variables, known and unknown, that come into play to be able to make any definitive proclamations. But I'll tell you this: Any road you travel down, you can turn around and travel back the other way. If you're unwell, the path you took to arrive at your present state of health can be traveled in the other direction. What I'm saying is that any illness that has not yet caused irreparable harm can absolutely be reversed. How that is accomplished is what is open for debate.

I cannot say that the information in this book will reverse existing problems for you . . . but it might. There is only one way to find out. If what you read resonates with you on a deep level, and your common sense calls out that it sounds logical and reasonable, then try it and see if you are one of the ones for whom it has been the right course of action. Whatever you do, never ever give up your faith in the supreme, unparalleled intelligence at work in every cell of your body. We've all heard of "miracle" healings. If it can happen once, it can happen more than once.

Now I want to ask you a question—a question that you need to ask of yourself. What are you willing to do to support your body's effort to attain the highest level of health available to you? Knowing that your body, with the brain at its helm, is tirelessly working for you, doing everything and anything it can to keep you in health, are you willing to also make an effort to help? Or are you of a mind that you want to just go your merry way and leave it all up to fate? I think when you see how simple the three CARE principles are, how much sense they make, and how easy they are to incorporate into your lifestyle, you will be excited about at least trying them. Well . . . turn the page and I'll show you how you can do exactly that.

ELEVEN

The First Principle: Periodic Monodieting

All three CARE principles, each working in concert with one another, are important, and all will help you immensely in your effort to live a life free of pain and disease, which is the automatic result of living a lifestyle that prevents cells from being driven crazy. But the first principle, periodic monodieting, if practiced intelligently, will do more to cleanse and strengthen your lymph system than any other action you could take besides fasting.*

More than any other factor, periodic monodieting is, without question, responsible for my recaptured health and my con-

---

*The subject of fasting is far too complex and deserves far more space than can be allotted here. Suffice it to say, however, that there is no health routine that is more thorough, effective, or beneficial than a properly conducted fast, and no other area of healing that is more neglected, misunderstood, or unfairly maligned. Those who call fasting and starvation the same thing are sorely ignorant of the physiology of the human body. It would be like calling swimming and drowning the same thing.

tinued well-being. I have benefited immeasurably from the practice for thirty years and continue to reap the rewards of its effectiveness in helping me maintain the level of health I enjoy. The beauty of periodic monodieting is its simplicity. Anyone can make use of this tool to bring about an immediate improvement in health and to ensure long-term health. It is the key element in preventing ill health while nurturing vibrant health.

WHAT IS PERIODIC MONODIETING?

Periodic monodieting is the eating of fresh fruits and/or vegetables and their juices, uncooked, for a length of time that ranges from one day to several weeks. Before explaining the rationale of monodieting and the benefits that can be expected from it, let me give you three examples of possible monodiets.

1. Drinking only fresh fruit and vegetable juice for 1 to 3 days.
2. Drinking only fresh fruit and vegetable juices and eating whole fruits and vegetables for 3 to 5 days.
3. Drinking only fresh fruit and vegetable juices and eating only fresh fruits and vegetables and salads for 1 day to a week to 10 days.

In other words, periodic monodieting is the taking of any combination of any raw, fresh food or juice for whatever length of time you wish.

The reason that all food during a monodiet must be in its natural, raw state is quite simple, and crucial to the cleansing of the lymph system.

PURPOSES OF MONODIETING

The purpose of monodieting is twofold. The first purpose is to use as little energy as possible on digestion so that energy can be freed and directed toward the cleansing and rejuvenation of the lymph system. The second purpose of monodieting is to obtain the maximum amount of fuel and nutrients from the food being eaten. Raw food fulfills these two purposes of monodieting better than cooked or processed food. Raw food demands less energy to digest and provides the most nutrients because it is in its purest state, its natural state. *Any* cooking of food removes or denatures some nutrients. Bear in mind that human beings are the only species that eats cooked food, and humans lead all species in degenerative diseases. Obviously our superior thinking and reasoning abilities have not served us in this area.

Ideally, periodic monodieting should not be used as a diet in a crisis to empty out a swollen lymph gland or to deal with an existing cancer, although in both instances the approach can and has been beneficial. To gain the greatest benefit from periodic monodieting, make it a regular part of your lifestyle and use it as a means of long-term prevention and long-term wellness. Remember: The extent to which you use periodic monodieting is up to you; there are an unlimited number of ways to use it, and there are no specifically prescribed regimens. Some people have an all-juice or all-fruit day once a week. Some eat only raw food one day a week. Some have three straight raw days every month. Author and lecturer Dr. Gabriel Cousens suggests that every six months you drink only fresh juices for a week. One doctor reports, "Short-term monodieting gives the weakened digestive system a rest. I use monodiets with great success in allergic individuals, who experience no allergic symptoms during the diet. The cleansing effect as well as the elimination of potential allergens gives the immune system a chance to revitalize its activities."

The object of periodic monodieting is, of course, to use it! If you must discipline yourself by marking on your calendar exactly when you are going to monodiet for a day or three days or five days or a week, then do it. Or if you wake up one morning and just feel like having only juice that day, then that's your day. Monodieting is a flexible tool; it's regimented only if you function better that way.

If I seem to be harping on this one aspect, it's because whenever food is discussed, people tend to look for restrictive rules they must follow as punishment for past dietary indiscretions. I encourage you to cultivate a different viewpoint, a new way of thinking. See periodic monodieting as a dynamic and integral part of your lifestyle that will bring you to a state of vibrant health and keep you there.

With periodic monodieting, the eating experience itself also becomes much more liberating. Moreover, one of the most rewarding results of monodieting, besides preventing disease, is the incredible surge of energy and well-being it produces. You will feel renewed and positive, and this feeling will spill over into every area of your life. Once you incorporate monodieting into your life, you never abandon it. Even if you monodiet only three days a year, you never get it out of your mind. You will look forward to monodieting with great anticipation because periodic monodieting is not a punishment, it is a joy!

Throughout the book I have made the point that the traditional approach to healing focuses solely on after-the-fact treatment. But the only way to prevent disease depends entirely upon what you do *before* such treatment is necessary. Periodic monodieting is the cornerstone of before-the-fact treatment, and therefore of a vibrant, healthy life.

When I embarked on my journey down the path to health, monodieting proved to be invaluable. At a time of desperate need, it gave me my first glimpse of how good I could feel. After starting with short monodiets of one, two, and three days, as my health steadily improved, I began increasing their duration until I was going ten days or two weeks, two or three times a year. My health problems dramatically improved, and I am convinced that periodic monodieting was the major reason for my recovery. To this day, it remains my most important tool for health maintenance.

The rationale behind periodic monodieting is simple as simple can be. The message of this book is that you can take charge of your health by cleansing the body of wastes and toxins. The means by which that is accomplished is to CARE— Cleanse and Rejuvenate Energetically. Periodic monodieting specifically and dramatically does just that. It greatly facilitates cleansing and skyrockets energy levels. And let's face it. Energy is everything. Without it, nothing is possible and nothing happens. A car without fuel goes nowhere; neither does a body without energy.

FREEING THE DIGESTIVE SYSTEM

There is no way on earth to discuss energy and energy levels without discussing digestion. When you take into account the full extent of the digestive activities involved in taking in food, processing it, extracting nutrients, and delivering them to the cells, the elimination of wastes and all the interactions of the organs, stomach, intestines, pancreas, liver, and kidneys, and the metabolic processes that turn food into blood, muscle, and bone, it is no wonder that the digestive process takes such an enormous amount of energy.

There is precious little you can do that requires more energy than digestion. You likely have evidence of this fact. After eating a big meal of many kinds of foods, for example, which do you look for, a mountain to climb or a sofa to climb onto? Knowing the extreme importance of energy to the cleansing process, what better place to free some than the vast amount required for digestion.

There are two ways to free energy from the digestive process for use in other areas of activity. The first is food combining, a concept I introduced in my previous books for just this purpose.

Allow me to review the basics of proper food combining for you. The two major food groups we eat are proteins (meat, chicken, eggs, fish, dairy) and starches (potatoes, rice, bread, pasta). Both proteins and starches are very concentrated foods requiring a significant energy output for digestion. Fruits and vegetables are not concentrated and so require far less energy for digestion.

When a protein enters the stomach, an acid-based digestive juice is required for digestion. When a starch enters the stomach, an alkaline-based digestive juice is required. Ever take a chemistry class? Do you know what happens when an acid and an alkaline come into contact with one another? They are neutralized. So, as an example, if you were to eat meat and potatoes, or fish and rice, or chicken and pasta, at the same meal, all combinations of a protein and a starch, the digestive juices are neutralized, causing the digestive process to be dragged out far too long.

Ever have a stomachache? How about acid indigestion or acid reflux? Or what about heartburn or gas pain? Or how about that heavy, bloated feeling after eating? All of these problems are the result of foods not being efficiently digested in the stomach. Rather, because they are forced to stay in the stomach for a prolonged length of time, the food starts to spoil, causing the above-listed discomforts. The two biggest-selling prescription drugs the world has ever known are Tagamet and Zantac. Both are for stomach disorders. Why do you think Americans spend billions upon billions of dollars every year for over-the-counter digestive aids? Because the digestive process has been severely thwarted by the combining of proteins and starches at the same meal.

The solution couldn't be simpler. If you want to eat a protein, have it with vegetables and salad, no starch. If you want to eat a starch, have it with vegetables and salad, no protein. That's it.

Literally tens of thousands of people have contacted me to tell me that they suffered from all manner of digestive pains for years on end before properly combining proteins and starches. Now they have no discomfort whatsoever, without drugs! I'm one of them. The more streamlined the digestive process, the less pain and discomfort. It's that simple.

"Food combining is imperative for sick patients," says one doctor. "I advocate food combining to insure that patients get a high intake of nutrients. Its helps them avoid the negative effects of maldigestion which plague so many sick people. Food combining doesn't overtax the already overstressed digestive tract and allows for the proper elimination of toxins or undigested food particles in the gut."

Want absolute, unequivocal proof? Try eating proteins and starches in the manner described, and in one week or less you'll have all the proof you'll ever need. You can become one of the millions of people who have discovered how well they can feel after eating, with no drugs for dessert. For an in-depth explanation and discussion of proper food combining, please check out the original *Fit for Life*.

The second way to free huge amounts of energy, is to give the digestive tract less to do. With less work to do, energy that is routinely spent on digestion is automatically used by the body to cleanse itself of waste. The body always works on priorities, and removing impactions and silted-up waste that are interfering with the smooth operation of the system is right up on top of the list. Lymph nodes will not become swollen with waste if wastes in the body are kept to a minimum.

Thus, by giving the digestive tract less to do, periodic mono-dieting becomes probably the most compelling and potent tool you can use to prevent ever becoming sick. I know what a provocative and bold statement that is. Indeed, many people would immediately demand proof. Therefore, although the greatest proof of all is in the doing, let me offer a couple of exhibits, one scientific, the other observational.

Roy Walford is a medical doctor. He has been a UCLA professor since 1966 and is one of the world's most eminent gerontologists. The director of a sixteen-member research laboratory at UCLA for the study of immunology and the aging process, he was also a member of the White House Conference on Aging and the National Academy of Sciences Committee on Aging, as well as chairman of the National Institute on Aging Task Force in Immunology. He has written five books on immunology and aging and is a world-renowned expert in his field.

Dr. Walford has conducted numerous long-term experiments on aging. To be sure, his experiments have not focused on periodic monodieting, which is a term I have coined. But his experiments have studied the effect of less work for the digestive tract, over a long term, on health and longevity. Dr. Walford's findings fully substantiate my premise that the less work the digestive tract has to do, the healthier you will be and the longer you will live.

Dr. Walford's experiments with mice is what has contributed so greatly to his notoriety. Whereas the normal lifespan of mice is about two years, Dr. Walford's mice all live more than twice that long. If we humans could do that, we would be living beyond 150. It gets better. Not only do his mice all live twice as long as the norm, but amazingly, those that do develop heart disease or cancer, do so in significantly lower rates. Plus, the small number of mice that do develop these diseases, do so at a much later age than the mice living half as long. And how has he managed to accomplish this extraordinary feat? He simply fasts his mice for two days a week. That's it. No drugs, no pills or potions, no shots, no magical formulas. A complete rest of the digestive tract for two days a week *doubles* their lifespan and reduces the incidence of disease. There's actually less disease in the mice living twice as long. Brothers and sisters—that's impressive. Dr. Walford is in his seventies and he fasts two days a week.[221]

The doctor's experiments support what practitioners of Natural Hygiene have known for a long while: that consuming food, using what is needed, and ridding itself of the rest will take more energy from the body over a lifetime than any other activity. Learning to channel some of that energy toward cleansing that will ultimately result in vibrant health is a gift of immeasurable value. That is the gift of periodic monodieting.

The practice of giving the digestive tract less work to do in order to free energy for the healing process is common throughout nature. Anyone who has worked a farm or spent time working with animals has seen this over and over. A horse that is lame will "go off its feed," as the expression goes. It will hardly eat. Every stockyard worker knows that when day after day a cow or horse or hog or sheep eats much less food than normal, there is something wrong with the animal. It has *instinctively* reduced its food intake so that its body will have the energy to correct whatever is wrong. Pet owners know that when their dog or cat is sick or injured, the animal either refuses food altogether or hardly eats at all. Even when concerned owners try to entice their sick pets with the most tempting food, the animal will refuse. They find a secluded spot and rest until the body completes its healing work. You've noticed this yourself, haven't you?

A similar reaction can be seen in children. When they are ill, they lose their appetite and won't eat. Parents frequently try to pressure them into eating by saying things like, "Eat this for Mommy," or, "The doctor says you won't get well if you don't eat." But having not been conditioned to believe that they have to eat when they're sick, they merely follow their instincts and refuse food. You have likely noticed a loss of appetite when you don't feel well. You recall my pointing out in the Seven Stages of Disease that loss of appetite is probably the single most obvious indicator of a body striving to cleanse and repair itself. That loss of appetite is a natural tendency of the body to free the energy from digestion that is needed for other work. And although monodieting is a smart thing to do to speed recovery when you're not feeling well, the most intelligent use of periodic monodieting—indeed its prime use and benefit—is as a normal and natural part of your lifestyle, as a means of preventing illness in the first place. It is an approach that will help you shift the focus from illness to wellness!

SCHEDULING YOUR MONODIET

I do not recommend that monodieting be used as an emergency measure (the same way you would use a drug) once the effect of continued neglect of the body has finally caught up to you. It should become a regular part of your healthy lifestyle, the same as anything else you do on a regular basis. Would you ever seriously consider not dusting and cleaning your house periodically? Would you ever dream of not periodically changing the old oil in your car? Then you mustn't consider not periodically monodieting to cleanse your inner body, because a clean inner body is easily as important—in fact, infinitely more important—than a clean house or car. Why? Because a clean inner body is what ensures your success in living a healthy life free of pain, ill health, and disease.

How can you find the monodieting option that is best for you? The only way to make an intelligent, informed decision on how and when to monodiet is to experience the benefits. Only then can you decide how and when to monodiet on a regular basis. While any amount of monodieting is beneficial, only on monodiets of three days and more do you really start to see the power behind this practice. But even a one-day monodiet will get you started and give you some idea of what to expect from future monodiets. With practice, it will become clear to you how to best incorporate monodieting into your lifestyle. Those whose lives are very orderly and regimented and who like knowing exactly when they are doing what will schedule their monodiets the same way they schedule other important events in their lives. Those who are more spontaneous will wake up one morning and declare, "I'm doing fruit and juice for three days." Neither approach is better than the other.

The following three monodiets—one day on juice; three days on juice, whole fruit, and smoothies; one week on only uncooked food—are examples only, not dictums. Follow them precisely or modify them to your likes and dislikes. The only hard-and-fast rule is: Nothing cooked.

ONE DAY ON JUICE

For one day, intermittently throughout the day, take in only juice, either fruit or vegetable or both. I have found that fruit juices work best for the first part of the day, with vegetable juice in the second part, and more fruit juice in the evening. But any way you want to do it is fine. You can have only fruit juice, only vegetable juice, or have fruit, then vegetable, back and forth throughout the day and evening. As long as it's only juice you're taking in, it doesn't matter which you have or when. Also, when having only juice, it's best to consume approximately 10 to 14 ounces about every 2 hours. Again, that is only a guideline; feel free to alter it to fit your particular needs and desires.

It is important that you consume only fresh juice for 24 hours. Many books on juicing will give you an amazingly wide array of different juice combinations, both fruit and vegetable. Experiment. These drinks are fun and they're delicious. One of my very favorites is apple-celery juice. "Ugh, apple-celery?" Right? Well, if you've never had it, you're in for a big surprise. Apple-celery juice is one of the most refreshing and delicious combinations I've ever had. There's something about that mixture that works. Just try it. You'll be hooked like so many other people I have turned on to it.

If you have read *Fit for Life,* you might be saying, "Hold on there, I thought it was a huge no-no to mix fruit with any other food." That is true, but like everything in life, there are exceptions to the rule. Since it is very high in water content and has no complex starches, proteins, or fats, celery causes no problem when eaten with fruit. But be warned: Celery juice is very potent; when combining it with apple juice, make the mixture approximately three-quarters apple juice, one-quarter celery juice.

THREE DAYS OF JUICE, WHOLE FRUIT, AND SMOOTHIES

On this monodiet, in addition to fresh juices throughout the day, you also eat pieces of fruit and fruit smoothies. Any fresh fruit is okay, and dried fruits such as dates and raisins are acceptable as long as they are dried naturally and do not contain sulphur dioxide. Dried fruit is very concentrated, so go lightly when having it.

Smoothies are extremely easy to make. Put either apple or orange juice (fresh, of course) in a blender, add a frozen banana and any other fruit you like, and presto, a fabulous smoothie. You can add frozen blueberries, strawberries, peaches, or other fruits to the juice and frozen banana. Have fun with these drinks. There are an infinite variety, and they taste incredible. (To freeze bananas, peel them first and put them in the freezer in an airtight plastic container.)

A WEEK ON ONLY UNCOOKED FOOD

For a week eat nothing but raw, uncooked food—all fruits and vegetables, their juices, and salads. Have as much juice and whole fruit and vegetables as you like and have a good-sized mixed salad late in the day with a salad dressing of olive oil (which has been associated with a significant reduced risk of cancer[222]), lemon juice, and your favorite herbs and spices. You can have other types of dressing, preferably with a minimum of chemical additives. After you consume the salad, refrain from eating fruit and fruit juice for three hours.

Remember, the above three monodiets are examples only. You could do any of them for any length of time. Number 1 could be done for several days or a week, as could Number 2. Or Number 3 could be done for one day or three. Or you could do Number 1 for a day, Number 2 for a day, and Number 3 for a day. Anything goes when monodieting in terms of duration as long as the fruits and vegetables eaten are uncooked.

TIPS AND TIDBITS FOR PERIODIC MONODIETING

1. For the most effective results of monodieting, the juices you drink must be fresh, not pasteurized, canned, or made from concentrate. Drinking other than fresh, unheated juice almost entirely defeats the purpose of monodieting. These days, home juicers are readily available and very reasonably priced. When measured against the benefits you will reap, the cost of a home juicer is insignificant. Owning your own juicer is a smart move. You probably have at least one television set in your house. Well, a juicer is a whole lot less expensive and has the added enticement of helping you prevent disease. Will your television set do that for you? If you don't own a juicer, buy fresh-squeezed juice. That will do fine. I've been using a Champion Juicer for thirty years. They are a bit more expensive (about $250), but they are extremely easy to use and clean, and are incredibly well made. I used the same Champion for over twenty years before replacing it. And the only reason I replaced it was because I wanted a different color.

2. When drinking juice, it is best not to gulp it down. Sip it instead. Drink it slowly so that all of it does not wind up in your stomach at once, which is hard on the body, can cause stomachaches, and is counterproductive. Swallow one mouthful at a time after the juice has had a chance to mix with your saliva.

3. Whether you are monodieting or not, you should not have fruit or fruit juice for about 3 hours after eating anything else. Fruit has a very interesting nature. Unlike other foods, fruit does not require a lot of time in the stomach for digestion. Most foods stay in the stomach about 3 hours. Fruit leaves the stomach in about 20 to 30 minutes. Fruit juice leaves the stomach in less time than that.

4. If you have never eaten highly cleansing food exclusively for a few days, you may experience a side effect that is uncomfortable but quite valuable: diarrhea. Understand that a certain amount of waste will accumulate in the digestive tract over time. When all of a sudden nothing but juice and fruit, which are over 90 percent water, suddenly goes through your system for a few days, it is as though the digestive tract is being flushed and scrubbed. Diarrhea will rarely last more than 48 hours, and usually will last only 24 hours. Remember, every action of the body is the result of a cause. After consuming only high-water, cleansing foods, diarrhea is not at all surprising. Of course, if you experience diarrhea for longer than 48 hours, for any reason, check with your health-care practitioner immediately. But to experience it because you're eating cleansing food is not something to be alarmed about.

5. Because their intake of food is so restricted while monodieting, some people think that they may not have enough energy to work or do other things they need to do. Interestingly, the opposite is true. Your energy levels will soar when you monodiet. Remember that digestion requires huge

amounts of energy. Since you are eating only uncooked food, you are eating the foods that require the least amount of energy to digest but that supply a great deal of energy. The one thing people comment on when they monodiet more than anything else, is the enormous increase in energy they experience.

6. One of the first concerns that come to mind for those who have never eaten only uncooked food for any length of time is, "But I'll be so hungry eating like that. I won't be able to function if I'm hungry all the time." It is a totally understandable and legitimate concern, but one that is not borne out.

Have you ever experienced this particular scenario? You sit down to a nice meal, you eat everything on your plate because it happens to be something you enjoy eating, and you're completely full and satisfied at the end of the meal. Then, 45 minutes later, even though your stomach is still full from the meal eaten, you find yourself rooting around in the kitchen for something to eat. You don't even know why, and may be thinking something like, "What am I doing here? I'm not even hungry—I just ate." But still you have to have something. Sound familiar? If this is a scene that has been played out in your life in the past, you'll be pleased to learn that there is a totally understandable, physiologically sound explanation, as there is for all activities of the human body.

At the base of the brain there is a little mechanism called the appestat, which controls the appetite. The appestat is constantly monitoring the body, checking to be sure there are sufficient nutrients in the system. If there are, the appestat is silent. If there are not sufficient nutrients, then the appestat sounds an alarm that tells us: "Let's eat!" And that alarm is not silenced until we eat the nutrients needed by the body. Sadly, however, there are those who eat when their appestat prods them to do so, but the food, because of cooking and processing, is so denatured and devoid of nutrients that the appestat just keeps on sounding the alarm. So, even though the stomach is full, those people are still "hungry"—not for food, but for nutrients. But all the body knows is that it is being encouraged to eat more so as to bring in the required nutrients. So, there we are in the kitchen with our full stomachs looking for some snack to eat because as far as the body is concerned, it hasn't been fed yet.

When monodieting, you are consuming foods that are brimming over with nutrients. Nothing has been degraded, destroyed, or removed. From the body's perspective, it's as though it won the lottery. When for several days in a row (or for however many days), the body is treated to foods that have not been altered in any way from their natural state, the body is flooded with high-quality, immediately available nutrients that saturate the system. Under these circumstances the appestat has no need to sound the alarm that in effect says, "Time to eat!"

7. People who are prone to hypoglycemia (low blood sugar) get a little nervous about eating only fruit or eating very lightly. Well, let's examine what low blood sugar is. The brain constantly monitors the bloodstream to make sure there is sufficient sugar (and other nutrients) in the blood. If there is an insufficient supply, the brain sets off an alarm in the form of edginess, discomfort, and sluggishness. Fruit, whose sugar component of fructose turns to glucose, goes into the bloodstream faster than anything else. So if you have low blood sugar, eating fruit will stop the symptoms of hypoglycemia very quickly. There's nothing better for low blood sugar than fruit. But people with hypoglycemia have to eat quite frequently to stem the symptoms. No problem. When monodieting, if you have hypoglycemic tendencies, you can eat as frequently as you feel you need to.

8. The word "sugar" is like a two-sided coin. On the one hand, sugar, in its *natural* state, is arguably the most important food of all for humans, because that's the only thing the body burns for energy (glucose). So important is glucose for life that

even if not supplied with sufficient amounts of carbohydrates (which are transformed into glucose), the body has a built-in mechanism to use fat reserves and turn them into glucose, and can actually, if need be, turn protein to glucose (gluconeogenesis).

On the other hand, processed and refined sugar is a deadly, virulent poison and has been associated with so many different diseases and metabolic disturbances that it would be difficult to discuss them all.

The absolute finest, most health-supporting and beneficial sugar you can consume is fructose, the energy component in fruit. It is so easily and efficiently utilized by the body that it does not even require digestion. It is absorbed directly into the body, primarily in the liver, and is converted into glucose during that absorption process. It is then available for immediate fuel needs or stored in the liver as glycogen for later energy use. That's why it's the most natural thing in the world to have a "sweet tooth." Unfortunately over the last 200 years "refined" sugars have gradually replaced the natural sugars in our diet and we are paying a dear price.

Refining means to make "pure" by a process of extraction or separation. Sugars are refined by taking a natural food that contains a high percentage of sugar and then removing all elements of that food until only the sugar remains.

White sugar is commonly made from sugar cane or sugar beets. Through heating and mechanical and chemical processing, all vitamins, minerals, proteins, fats, enzymes, and indeed, *every* nutrient is removed. Sugar cane and sugar beets are first harvested and then chopped into small pieces, squeezing out the juice, which is then mixed with water. This liquid is then heated and lime is added. Moisture is boiled away, and the remaining fluid is pumped into vacuum pans to concentrate the juice. By this time, the liquid is starting to crystallize and is ready to be placed into a centrifuge machine where any remaining residues are spun away. The crystals are then heated to the boiling point and are passed through charcoal filters.

After the crystals condense, they are bleached snow white usually by the use of cattle bones.

During these refining processes, sixty-four food elements are destroyed. All the potassium, magnesium, calcium, iron, man-ganese, phosphate, and sulfate are removed. The A, B, and D vitamins are eliminated. Amino acids, vital enzymes, unsaturated fats, and all fiber are gone.

When you eat a refined carbohydrate like sugar, the body must take vital nutrients from healthy cells to metabolize the incomplete food. Sodium, potassium, magnesium, and calcium are drawn from various parts of the body to make use of the sugar. So much calcium is used to neutralize the effects of sugar that the bones, which are the body's storehouse of this mineral, become osteoporotic due to the withdrawn calcium. The teeth are likewise affected, and they lose their components until decay occurs and hastens their loss. So not only does sugar provide no needed nutrients, it causes the body to rob itself of its own vital elements!

This refined sugar offal is being sneaked into your food in mind-boggling amounts. Right now over 150 pounds of re-fined sugar for every man, woman, and child in the United States are being produced every year. Read those labels. When you see words like sucrose, fructose, dextrose, turbinado, corn syrup or high fructose corn syrup, raw sugar, brown sugar, or molasses, as far as your body is concerned, they are, one and all, poisons.

These names may seem benign but do you really understand what they mean?

Guess what brown sugar is. Plain old superrefined white sugar with some molasses thrown in for color. So-called "raw sugar" is just white sugar that's missing one of the many refin-ing steps that all sugars go through, as is turbinado. I know I told you that fructose is the finest, most perfect sugar of all, but that's when it's obtained from fresh, nonprocessed fruit. Once processed, it's as bad as white sugar.

When sugar is being refined as described above, all the

chemicals and deranged nutrients, the waste by-products of the refining process, are collected. Rather than throwing it in some dump where it belongs, *it's added to your food!* It's called molasses. Yup, you read it right. Molasses is nothing more or less than the waste by-products of sugar refinement.

All of this poison in the guise of something sweet is being unloaded into your food. It's everywhere, even in certain "healthy" foods; just when you think you're doing something good for yourself, you're actually compromising your health. All of those fancy teas and the bottled "fruit" drinks that have become so popular have several teaspoons of some processed, refined sugar. Do you know those "fruit at the bottom" yogurt cups have 9 teaspoons of sugar? Nine! That's only one less teaspoon than a12-ounce can of cola. And here you thought it was a health food.

All I can say is, be careful, be aware. Make a good-faith effort to cultivate a taste for the real thing: fresh fruit. I'm not suggesting you never eat anything with refined sugar in it, that's not very realistic. But be in the know. Cut back when you can and your body will thank you in so many ways. The two books I read that blew the lid off the sugar conspiracy were *Sugar Blues* by William Dufty and *Sweet and Dangerous* by John Yudkin. Another great book on the subject written more recently is *Sugar Busters* by H. Leighton Steward et al.

9. When monodieting on all raw, uncooked food, many people like to eat nuts. It's okay to eat raw nuts when monodieting; however, you have to be careful. Nuts are an *extremely* concentrated food that is exceedingly easy to overeat. They should be eaten very sparingly, and not more than once a day. Ten or twelve almonds, for example, are plenty. More than that makes your digestive tract work too hard, exactly what you want to avoid. If you can't eat only ten or twelve nuts, leave them alone.

Also, whenever I eat nuts (I am partial to raw almonds and raw cashews), I always have either cucumber slices or celery with them. Not only does the combination taste great, but the high water content of the cucumbers and celery seems to assist in moving the nuts through the stomach more easily. You may question the wisdom of eating nuts at all because of their fat content. As we have discussed, however, some fat in the diet is absolutely essential. Without some fat, you would die. In fact, vitamins A, D, E, and K cannot be broken down and used unless they are in the presence of fat. The issue is where the fat in your diet is coming from. The fat in animal products is the culprit, not the fat from raw nuts and seeds, or avocados.

10. If you monodiet for a week or longer on all uncooked foods—salads, in addition to juices, fruit, smoothies, and vegetables—you may start to crave something cooked, but still want to continue your monodiet. Adding some steamed vegetables to your salad allows you to continue to cleanse but also to eat a little more heavily. Choose whatever vegetables you like: broccoli, cauliflower, zucchini, etc. Steam one, two, or three, put them in your salad, add dressing and *voilà,* an incredibly tasty and satisfying meal.

Don't add steamed vegetables on short monodiets of only three or four days. But if you're going for a week or two weeks, add steamed veggies for the last part of the monodiet. In other words, on a one-week monodiet, add steamed vegetables the last two days. On a ten-day monodiet, add steamed vegetables the last three or four days. Also, make sure there is more salad than steamed vegetables, not the other way around. Remember, it is the regular eating of *uncooked* food that is the goal.

11. A beautiful side effect of periodic monodieting is that your overall diet tends to improve. After eating clean, healthful food for a while, you're not so willing to put just anything in your body. Sometimes the change is obvious, sometimes it's subtle, but as time goes by and you are free of pain, you've lost weight, your energy is up, and you're feeling very good about

yourself, you'll want to keep it that way. You'll find yourself making healthier menu choices in restaurants and eating those death-burgers and fries less frequently at the thousands of fast-food places that contribute so greatly to the level of ill health suffered by so many.

12. After ending a monodiet of five days or longer, be particularly careful of what you eat for a day or two. Eating a lot of very heavy foods too quickly can make you feel horrible. Your body accustoms itself to light, clean, uncooked food and you can catch it off guard by too quickly eating too heavily. Let's say you do a one-week monodiet of juices, fruit, and salads. If on the eighth day you consume a big lunch of pizza or fried chicken or a burger and fries and a dinner of steak and potatoes, bread, and apple pie, you're going to feel miserable the next day. It would be better to eat very lightly in the morning, only fruit and/or juice. Have a salad and a baked potato for lunch or a piece of toast if you need more than salad, and perhaps a pasta-with-vegetable dish and a salad for dinner. This way you gradually reintroduce the cooked food without jumping straight into consuming the heaviest foods possible. Wait until the second or third day after a monodiet before having meat, chicken, or fish, and eat them sparingly (more on that in the next principle).

13. This tip is of such importance that I considered making it the fourth principle. It has to do with what foods you eat in the morning hours. I know that Americans have been raised to believe that a "big hearty breakfast" is the best way to start the day, but it ain't necessarily so.

To date, the Fit for Life books *(Fit for Life* and *Fit for Life II)* have sold over eleven million copies worldwide. Nearly half a million people have written to share their thoughts, ask questions, and make comments on these books and the principles they impart. Without question, the comment made far and away more frequently than any other, concerns what foods should be eaten in the early part of the day to ensure optimal health. I want very briefly to summarize that information for you here.

What we are trying to accomplish is a cleansing of your body—the elimination of waste—so that the lymph system will not be so overburdened that it has to store those toxic wastes in the lymph nodes, thereby opening the door for disease. Every physiological function of your body operates under cycles that are called circadian rhythms. The eight-hour period that the body's internal eliminative processes are most heightened is from 4:00 a.m. until 12 noon. That is when the lymph system is most active in picking up waste from the cells and taking them to the eliminative organs.

As discussed earlier, digestion takes enormous amounts of energy, so if you eat a heavy meal in the morning hours, some of the energy being used to cleanse and eliminate is diverted to the stomach for digestion. To get the absolute most from the three principles, eat as lightly as possible in the hours from the time you awaken in the morning until noon. If you can eat exclusively fruit and juice until noon, as much as you like, that is certainly the very best routine possible, because fruit and its juices require practically no energy at all to be digested. That way, the elimination cycle can operate at its fullest efficiency.

If you don't feel you can eat only fruit and juice until noon, try the following two suggestions:

- Eat only fruit and its juices until noon as often as you can. If that's only two days a week, so be it. If it's every other day, that's fantastic.
- At least make fruit and juice the first thing you put into your body, even if a half hour later you're having cereal and toast.

The goal should be to go as close to noon as you can on only fruit and juice. You'll need only one week to see the phenomenal difference that eating fruit until noon makes in your energy level and feeling of well-being. Millions have already learned about it, have made it a permanent part of their lives, and are enjoying the many benefits of the practice. The results will astound you. In terms of experiencing your highest level of health, this tip is very important for your overall success. Please do not minimize it. (Refer to *Fit for Life* for an in-depth explanation of circadian rhythms and the value of consuming fruit until noon.)

14. A question you are sure to ask is: "How often should I monodiet and for how long?" Generally speaking, if you have never monodieted or fasted, or taken any other measures to cleanse or detoxify your system, and you are fairly certain your inner body could use a good cleansing, the more frequent and the longer the monodiet, the better. In other words, at first, diligently monodiet at regular intervals; later, your monodiets will be more for maintenance, especially if you upgrade your diet by minimizing foods that would encumber your lymph system.

The best illustration I can give you is my own experience with monodieting. When I was introduced to Natural Hygiene and monodieting, I was highly motivated. I was sick, fat, tired, in pain, and living in fear because of the death of my father, as a result of cells being driven crazy in his body. The person who taught me the fundamentals of monodieting assured me that a series of monodiets and simultaneous improvement in my dietary habits would quickly bring me to a level of health I had not enjoyed for a very long time.

Let me tell you, he sounded totally sure of himself and I sorely wanted to believe. But for as long as I had been dealing with excruciating stomachaches, for as many weight-loss diets as I had been on, for as frustrated as I was over my continually declining health, I have to admit that I was more than a little skeptical that it would all be wiped away by what seemed to be hardly any effort. But there was something else. I was willing!

My mentor told me that the first thing I needed to do, since I was eating anything I desired at any time, was to have only fruit and vegetable juices and fresh fruit for five days. At that particular stage of my life, the idea of eating only fruit and juices for five days was like suggesting that I wet my finger and stick it in a light socket. But I did what my mentor advised because I desperately needed something to turn things around for me. The first day was the hardest. The first day is always the hardest. But on the sixth day, when I was supposed to start eating other foods, the most amazing, most unexpected thing happened: I felt so darned good, so energetic, so positive, so light and clean, that I decided to go for another five days! Me! The guy who would rather fall down a flight of concrete stairs than miss a meal.

I was riding my bicycle every day and reading books by Herbert M. Shelton, the acknowledged father of Natural Hygiene. At the end of ten days, my life was forever changed. I simply could not believe how good I felt. My stomach, which had hurt every day for more than 20 years, did not bother me at all, I had lost about 12 pounds, my energy level was through the roof, and I felt as if I owned the world.

My mentor, who had a rather quirky sense of humor, said to me, in a totally professional, serious tone, "Well, you have a decision to make now. You can either alter your dietetic lifestyle a bit and continue to cleanse your system, lose more weight, and feel euphoric, or you can go back to the way you were eating before your ten days and have your health go back to what it was. What's it going to be?" I didn't say anything, I just looked at him in a way that left no doubt what my decision was.

He told me that for the best results, the quickest results, I should cut out all meat, at least at first. Then after I felt really good, I could reintroduce the meat into my diet, but not the way I was eating it before, which was not only every day, but every meal.

I decided to eliminate all meat, chicken, and fish from my diet at least until I lost 50 pounds. I basically ate whatever I wanted other than those foods, being sure not to overeat.

Although I ate breads, cheese, pasta, and the like, fruits and vegetables dominated my diet. I monodieted two days a week, one day on juices only (fruit and vegetable) and another day (three days later) on juice and whole fruit, as much as I liked.

Astonishingly, I lost the 50 pounds in one month. Not only was my body ready to heal itself, I also helped it along by improving my diet, riding my bike every day, and flooding my consciousness with positive thoughts about how well I was doing and how successful I was going to be.

I made a commitment to do a ten-day monodiet at least four times a year, one every three months. For the next two years, I did exactly that—every three months I did either ten days on juices and fruit or ten days on juice, fruit, and salads. In between, I ate very few animal products, exercised regularly, and did shorter monodiets of one or two days in a row every week. After the first two years, with my weight loss maintained, no pain, and an exuberance for life that I thought I'd never achieve, I knew I had found a lifestyle that would serve me forever. Now I do ten-day monodiets two or sometimes three times a year, and I monodiet one or two days a week.

I tried different kinds of monodieting routines. Once I ate only uncooked foods (fruit, vegetables, juice, and salads) every other day for three months. In between, I ate what I wanted. It was great! I felt absolutely incredible. When I was preparing for my first television tour to promote *Fit for Life*, I ate only fruit and juices for two weeks and only uncooked food for a month. Touring is unbelievably grueling, but I sailed through three weeks of nonstop work with interviews from morning until night and a plane ride every day, with an abundance of energy and positive feelings. Over and over, television talk-show hosts would comment on how "up and energetic" I was for being in the middle of a tour.

So let's get back to your original question: "How often should I monodiet and for how long?" My advice is to start with a three- or five-day monodiet of fruit and vegetable juices and whole fruit, just to see what it feels like. Then monodiet one or two days a week, every week, and a week to ten days every three to four months, depending on how much cleansing you feel your body needs and how motivated you are to get your lymph system cleaned out so that no lymph nodes become encumbered with waste. As I've said above, the duration and frequency of your monodiet is up to you.

Having said that, I know some of you prefer to follow a more definitive program—something that removes the guesswork. Once again, a quick analogy: If you were in a canoe or a rowboat that had a lot of water in it because of a leak, you would have to bail aggressively to lower the water level and prevent capsizing. Once you reduced the level of water, you could relax and bail only periodically to keep the water level low. So it is with your body. To start, you should monodiet more frequently and for longer durations, to lower the level of toxins in your body. Then you can monodiet more infrequently as a means to keep the level of toxins low.

For the first year, monodiet for at least ten days every three months. That's four ten-day monodiets for the year. Two should comprise only juice (both fruit and vegetable) and fruit, and two should be all raw foods (fruits, vegetables, their juices and salads). In between the ten-day monodiets, monodiet at least two days a week, either two days in a row or twice within the week. After the first year, you could continue the same pattern every year for the rest of your life, to be absolutely certain that your body's toxic level never gets out of control and your lymph nodes never become swollen, but as a maintenance program you can cut it in half. That would be two ten-day monodiets a year and at least one day a week.

Understand this: You cannot monodiet too much! The more you do it, the healthier you'll be and the likelihood of your ever driving cells crazy will diminish. You can, however, monodiet too little. Therefore, you have to find out what your personal comfort level is and how motivated you are. As time goes by, you will know exactly how much you need to monodiet for your particular lifestyle, especially when you experience the well-being that is the automatic result of regular periodic monodieting. Don't overthink about it. Jump in and do one and you will quickly see that it is not nearly the daunting challenge you may be thinking it is.

15. This last tip is one that I implore you to pay close attention to. The expressed purpose of periodic monodieting is to cleanse toxins from your body so they do not cause harm and eventually disease. Simply put, toxins are poisons, and when they are being removed from the body, they can, on occasion, cause distress, anything from mild uneasiness all the way to extreme discomfort. It would be marvelous if I could say that all you have to do is monodiet a few times and all the transgressions of the past will be washed away as you skip joyfully into the sunset in exuberant health—and quite often it is exactly like that. But sometimes, depending on all manner of variables that can come into play, it's uncomfortable and there's no getting around that.

It can happen that the very condition you suffer from, whether headaches or a skin condition or what have you, become more acute before it becomes better. What I want you to know is that as the body cleanses itself, the very thing you're trying to heal first becomes more pronounced. You may experience some real rip-snortin' headaches. Or your skin condition may become really bothersome. Now, as unpleasant as that sounds, it's health in action. It's health returning. And it is most definitely temporary. It is essential that you are clear on that. It proves that the monodieting is working, evidenced by the increased eliminative activity that is causing the discomfort. I wouldn't want you to make the effort, go on a monodiet for a few days, and then instead of feeling wonderful right away, feel lousy and quit with a, "Well, that didn't work, it just made things worse."

This discomfort I'm referring to doesn't happen all the time—not by a long shot—but it does happen. From experience, I can tell you that perseverance, faith, and trust go a long way. Stick to it and see it through if you experience discomfort. Have faith in the unparalleled recuperative powers of the human body. And trust that the infinite intelligence and wisdom that govern your body are working perfectly for your greater good. When the cleansing activities of the body that are causing the discomfort are completed, you will get to enjoy the feeling of renewal that is the automatic result of patiently allowing the dynamics of the body to do what it does best: heal itself.

BENEFITS OF THE FIRST PRINCIPLE

When you are monodieting, you are allowing your body to be cleansed. You are cleaning and rejuvenating your lymph system. *You are preventing disease.* Please, please do not make the mistake of taking periodic monodieting lightly or minimizing the extent to which it can achieve that much-desired goal of helping you live your life without the fear of becoming a medical statistic.

Considering the havoc that pain and disease have caused in so many people's lives and their apparently complicated and puzzling characteristics, I can understand your initial reaction being something like, "Yeah, right. Eating nothing but fruit and vegetables every so often is going to prevent diseases as pervasive and bewildering as cancer." Is there a problem with the solution being simpler and more straightforward than you have been led to believe? If it was far more complicated, expensive, and difficult to do, would you have more confidence in periodic monodieting then? Earlier, I told you about the woman who called me from the hospital because she had a walnut-sized lump in her breast. She got rid of the lump by monodieting! As far as she was concerned, monodieting saved her life.

For most of you, periodic monodieting is an aspect of your life that you have yet to experience. If for no other reason than curiosity, try it just to see what, if anything, you've missed. Having done so, you will certainly know your body better. When you buy a car or a VCR or a camera, don't you read the owner's manual to learn all about the item's features so you can use it to your best advantage? It would be great if our bodies came with an owner's manual, but that isn't the case. Still, don't you want to learn all about its features so that you can use it to its fullest and not miss out? Here is something that holds such great promise, and until now, the knowledge of it has somehow escaped you. Now is your chance to discover a part of you that you haven't known before.

If you own a fax machine or a computer, you've probably marveled at the way such machines have revolutionized our lives. You often hear people say such things as, "I don't know how in the world my business ran before fax machines." Or, "How on earth would I ever get by without my computer?" These are common expressions of those who have learned to depend heavily on modern technological wonders. Imagine how they would feel if suddenly they had to give them up. They would feel sorely deprived. It would be one thing if they had never experienced them and were not aware of the ways in which they could dramatically improve their lives, but to have them and use them and then lose them would be unbearable. And that is exactly what periodic monodieting is like. If you don't know what you're missing, then you don't know, and that's it.

However, once you discover firsthand how periodic mono-dieting can transform your health and, therefore, your life, you will never want to give it up. You mustn't allow the fact that monodieting is simple, inexpensive, and totally in your control to discourage you from trying it.

Ill health will be prevented only if you live a lifestyle that does not cause it. Making periodic monodieting a permanent part of your lifestyle is that certain "something" people have been looking for to finally win the battle over catastrophic disease and the years of pain and ill health that precede it.

Monodieting is a gift, a blessing, and once experienced, you'll
bless the day it became a part of your life.

A PERSONAL TESTIMONIAL

I feel compelled to share a personal story with you here
which should stand as a most impressive testimonial for periodic monodieting. In 1966, when I was twenty-one years old,
I was in the United States Air Force and sent to Vietnam for a
one-year tour of duty. While there, I was exposed to Agent
Orange and now have a condition called peripheral neuropa-
thy. All of the extensor muscles in both of my arms have atro-
phied. What that means is that I am unable to lift my arms
unless my palms are facing upward or unless I point my
elbows out to the sides first. I have a good grip in my hands but
I am unable to open them back up on their own. I also have a
slight limp in both of my legs. These problems do not keep me
from doing anything I want to do, but I have to use both of my
hands for the most simple of movements that even a small
child could accomplish with one hand.

Agent Orange, a derivative of dioxin, is one of the deadliest
chemicals ever formulated, and works in a very odd way in
that the deterioration of muscles that it inevitably causes begins approximately twenty years after exposure. I was exposed
in 1966 and my muscles started to deteriorate in 1986.

Having been in touch with the Agent Orange Support Group
in the United States, I've learned that thousands of individuals
who were exposed while in Vietnam are dealing with the same
thing as I. With one huge difference. It turns out that Agent
Orange just continues spreading throughout the body, and five
years after deterioration starts, individuals are either severely
restricted in their movements, wheelchair-bound, or dead. But
not so with me. It has been fifteen years since the deterioration
started and it looks as if I've managed to stop it. How did I do
that? I was exposed in 1966, and I learned all about the lymph

system and the need to clean it out on a regular basis in 1970. Although I had no idea that I was exposed to Agent Orange until my arms started to wither in 1986, four years after my exposure I started to periodic monodiet on a very regular basis for other reasons and that practice, it turns out, saved my life!

The reason I'm telling you this should be glaringly obvious. If periodic monodieting can save me from something as deadly as Agent Orange coursing through my veins, do you see what an exceedingly powerful tool it can be in your life? I pray that you do. If I can make headway with one of the deadliest chemicals ever produced, imagine what you could do if you were to start using periodic monodieting *before* you have a crisis on your hands. And that, my friend, is truly the meaning of prevention: taking steps while you are well, to see to it that you stay that way.

As far as I am concerned, I am alive and able to share life-saving information like this with others, thanks to periodic monodieting. Whatever you do, do not take lightly what you are learning here. As regards your well-being and longevity, periodic monodieting may very well be the most important tool you ever learn about. It certainly has been for me!

TWELVE

The Second Principle: The Gradual Reduction of Animal Products

In the previous chapter, you learned about the disease-preventing benefits of periodic monodieting. There are numerous other benefits associated with cleansing the inner body. As you become more familiar and more comfortable with the practice, these will become increasingly apparent. One of the subtler side effects is the body's natural inclination to consume less of those foods that clog it with the most toxic waste and require the greatest amount of energy to digest and eliminate.

As you might guess from what you've already read in this book, the food category that fits this description most accurately is animal products. Considering the fat, cholesterol, hormones, pesticides, antibiotics and other chemical and pharmaceutical contaminants, uric acid and bacterial putrefaction and contamination animal products contain, it's hard to come up with a food more responsible for toxifying the body with harmful wastes. Moreover, animal products are also the most structurally complex and difficult foods to break down in the body, thereby requiring more energy to process than any other. Add to this that animal products are devoid of fiber and are associated with every major disease that afflicts the population, and you have more than ample reason to actively seek out ways of cutting down on them in your diet. However, although these days people generally know that animal products are no longer the "celebrity" foods they use to be, and although authorities the world over recommend diets that deemphasize animal products, there is still that nagging voice at the back of your mind that may be telling you that protein is an important nutrient and protein means meat and other animal products.

THE BIG PROTEIN MYTH

So before presenting you with a simple, comfortable, workable strategy for reducing the amount of animal products in your diet, I think it's important to give you at least a brief bit of background on some of the reasons why you hold these not-so-healthy foods in such high regard.

Many of the disease statistics in America are the result of a deliberate campaign waged by the industries that would profit from our ignorance. For decades we've been pummeled with an avalanche of one-sided information pushing an animal-based point of view called the "Four Food Groups," half of which just happen to be animal products. This was done for profit, not health.

Interestingly, the idea that animals supply us with the finest source of protein can be traced back to studies on rodents that showed rats fare better on an animal-based diet than on a plant-based diet. [223] From these studies on rats, researchers jumped to the conclusion that animal protein was superior to plant proteins—for humans! Now, that is a jump that can only be compared to leaping across the Grand Canyon in a single bound in a heavy thunderstorm with both legs in a cast, because physiologically and anatomically we are very different from rats.

The animal products industries, however, ran with the rat research and promoted it to the outer reaches of the universe. These studies were later shown to be inapplicable to humans, in fact, ludicrous, because rats require a much more concentrated source of protein, such as meat, and their amino acids needs are different from those of humans. It was too late. The myth had been born and the animal products industries were hardly going to let it die.

DIETARY MODELS

In 1923, the United States Department of Agriculture (USDA) came up with the "Twelve Food Groups." Oddly, the Basic Twelve revolved around four diet plans that incorporated choices from each group and were structured to apply to different income brackets.[224] So protein could be obtained from the legumes (beans, lentils, split peas) and nuts category for lower-income individuals, or from the meat category for those who could afford higher-priced protein sources. Prestige was attached to animal products, because they were portrayed as preferred foods for the "upper" class. They were now "elitist foods." Long forgotten and extremely important to bear in mind is that it was never stated by the USDA that animal protein was superior to plant protein, only more expensive!

The Basic Twelve hung on until 1941, when the Food and Nutrition Board of the National Research Council, feeling that twelve were too cumbersome and difficult to remember, reduced the number to the "Seven Food Groups." Legumes and nuts were listed in the same category as meat, poultry, fish, and eggs. From the 1940s on, the National Egg Board, the National Dairy Council, and the National Livestock and Meat Board were running heavy campaigns praising the "ideal" protein in animal products.

By 1960, the now-famous (or infamous) "Four Food Groups" became the dominant dietary model in the country. Fruits and vegetables, which could rightly have been two groups, were lumped together, and animal products, which could rightly have been one group, were separated into meat and dairy. Legumes and nuts were pushed out altogether as a named protein source! Animal products were now king of the mountain, representing 50 percent of our daily recommended dietary intake, thus appearing to be as important as everything else combined. The animal products industries, for reasons that hardly need explanation, were in nirvana.

THE CASE AGAINST ANIMAL PRODUCTS REVISITED

Ironically, at this same time, research funded by the National Dairy Council uncovered the link between increased blood cholesterol and dairy fat. Subsequent studies confirmed this link and verified the increased risk of heart disease when cholesterol levels were increased. At the same time that dairy products were being pushed by the animal products industries, research was busily destroying the myth.

During the 1950s, more conclusive evidence that linked heart disease to the consumption of animal products came to light from a more unexpected source. During the Korean War, both American and Korean soldiers killed were autopsied. In the young Americans, with their high animal product intake, 77 percent already had narrowed blood vessels due to atherosclerotic deposits. No such damage appeared in the arteries of the equally young Koreans, whose national diet included far fewer animal products, with a higher vegetable and grain intake.[225]

At the same time, studies on Japanese individuals who had a long line of healthy hearts showed that those Japanese who moved to the United States and adopted the Western diet dominated by animal products had enormously higher rates of heart disease than their counterparts who stayed in Japan and consumed diets low in fat and cholesterol. By the early 1960s it was becoming apparent that there were some significant problems with the basic Four Food Group approach to diet.

As research increasingly began to prove conclusively that the consumption of animal products was harmful to health, the meat and dairy industries increased their efforts to encourage meat and dairy consumption. As the seventies rolled around, it became more and more difficult for the industries to pull this off because the evidence against the health benefits of consuming animal products started to rapidly build. The Senate Select Committee on Nutrition and Human Needs brought together many of the nation's most respected researchers, and their resulting recommendations reflected the increasingly conspicuous relationship between the American diet and disease. Their "alternative diet" deemphasized animal products and encouraged more selections from the plant kingdom. This was the first official statement that a move away from a meat-based diet would be an improvement to health!

In 1977, a follow-up to the panel's findings was released in a report entitled *Dietary Goals for the United States,* which supported the need for a new national diet and once again deemphasized animal products. The meat, dairy, and egg industries unleashed the pressure of the incredibly powerful cholesterol lobby and the original phrase in the report "eat *less* meat" was changed to "eat *lean* meat."[226] The original text of the report actually advised Americans to eat less meat in the mid-1970s, but the animal products industries were successful in pressuring legislators to keep that from you! How lovely.

The 1980s appeared to be as progressive in terms of improving the American diet as the 1970s, with further official recommendations instructing the public on the importance of minimizing their consumption of foods high in saturated fat and cholesterol (animal products). But right when everything was going along swimmingly, catastrophe struck. There was a political shift that very nearly sounded the death knell for nutritional reform.

The superpowerful animal food industries won out with the presidential election of 1984, after which efforts to continue educating the public were severely thwarted. In the words of Michael Jacobson, head of the Center for Science in the Public Interest, "When Ronald Reagan was elected President, the Department of Agriculture, the lead agency for nutritional education, was basically given over to the meat industry."[227]

Reagan's secretary of agriculture was a hog farmer. His deputy secretary had been president of the American Meat Institute for eight years. One of the assistant secretaries had been head of the National Cattlemen's Association, and the head of the Bureau of Land Management, the organization that decides how much public land would be given over to animal agriculture, was a Colorado cattleman. Not a moment was wasted in undoing advances that had been made in the effort to increase the public's knowledge about diet and health. Dissenting nutritionists were either silenced or fired.

Although the 1980s were not kind to nutritional education, they did end on a high note with the release of the Surgeon General's Report on Nutrition and Health, the report from the National Academy of Sciences, the heart and cancer associations' positions and urgings from other health-related organizations. *All* were imploring Americans to reduce their consumption of foods high in fat and cholesterol, specifically animal products.

So, here we are all primed to get on with the twenty-first century. Where do we stand with the Four Food Groups? To what extent is the government involved, either in terms of helping us or capitulating to the profit motive? These days there's hardly anyone who walks upright not aware of the dangers of consuming meat. When was the last time you read an obituary column full of the names of people who died due to an insufficient amount of fat and cholesterol in their arteries?

THE EATING RIGHT PYRAMID

This brings us to the most provocative story of the Four Food Group controversy to date. Thirty-five years of haggling and maneuvering to replace the Four Food "wheel" with something more in line with our actual needs finally came to a resolution in 1991. "The Eating Right Pyramid" (see the figure below) was unveiled by the USDA to replace the Four Food Groups "wheel." In this pyramid, although the actual recommended servings of each food group were not changed, the difference is in the visual presentation. The foods we are being encouraged to emphasize in our diets occupy the biggest space. Those foods that are harmful are no longer represented in 50 percent of the diagram. You see, the average number of servings of animal products recommended is five per day, whereas the average number of servings recommended of fruits, vegetables, and grains is fifteen per day, three times as many. So you can see that the wheel, which gave the visual impression that animal products were to be consumed in equal amounts to everything else combined, was totally misleading. The pyramid ingeniously rectified this glaring inconsistency.

Those foods which we should eat the most—grains and legumes—are on the broad bottom. Then, in ascending order by number of recommended servings, are fruit and vegetables, then animal foods, then fats, which are represented by the tip of the pyramid, along with the admonition to use sparingly. Brilliant!

But only days before its release date, like a bolt of lightning out of the blue, Agriculture Secretary Edward R. Madigan withdrew it. "But why?" you must be asking. Just prior to the release of the Eating Right Pyramid, Mr. Madigan had a private meeting with board members of the National Cattlemen's Association. A few days later, he received a letter from the American Meat Institute, and then the National Milk Producers Federation complained that dairy products were too

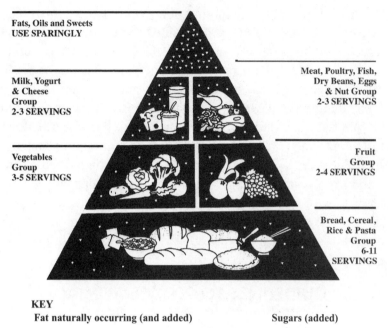

**Fats, Oils and Sweets
USE SPARINGLY**

**Milk, Yogurt
& Cheese
Group
2-3 SERVINGS**

**Meat, Poultry, Fish,
Dry Beans, Eggs
& Nut Group
2-3 SERVINGS**

**Vegetables
Group
3-5 SERVINGS**

**Fruit
Group
2-4 SERVINGS**

**Bread, Cereal,
Rice & Pasta
Group
6-11
SERVINGS**

KEY
Fat naturally occurring (and added)   Sugars (added)
These symbols show fat and added sugars in foods.

close to fat in the pyramid. The next thing we knew, the pyramid was out the window.[228] The Center for Science in the Public Interest released a statement that said, "The Department of Agriculture is just what the name says, the Department of Agriculture. It consistently puts the interests of the meat, egg, and dairy industries ahead of the public's health."[229]

In what can only come under the category of rubbing hot sauce into an already open wound, Mr. Madigan's highly suspect reason for withdrawing the pyramid was "because it had not been tested on children."[230] This didn't come to him until only moments before the release date of the pyramid and after three years of testing? He would have had fewer eyes rolling if he'd said that extraterrestrials came into his bedroom and warned that Earth would be destroyed if the Eating Right Pyramid was released!

Fortunately, in a rare but welcome victory for the beleaguered consumer, under tremendous pressure from an outraged health and nutrition community, the pyramid was reinstituted in 1992 and supplanted the antiquated food group wheel. The director of nutrition at the Center for Science in the Public Interest summed it up best when she said that the decision "shows that, at least sometimes, the public wins."[231] It's a funny thing about the truth, it doesn't go away. It can be stamped on, abused, distorted, corrupted, or buried, but like a balloon full of air that is pushed under water, it keeps popping back up. And the truth here is indisputable and undeniable. Notwithstanding the self-serving, greed-motivated propaganda from the animal products industries, we *must* start to reduce our consumption of animal products—the second principle of the CARE program—for many reasons other than preventing disease.

GUIDELINES TO REDUCE ANIMAL PRODUCT CONSUMPTION

Undoubtedly, there are many people who know that they should minimize consumption of animal-based products in their diets, and genuinely want to eat less of these foods, but they don't know how to accomplish their goal in a way that allows them to enjoy the eating experience without creating turmoil in their lives. The second principle is how. It provides you with an intelligent approach to gradually change your "eating style," a workable formula that shows you a specific plan of action rather than just saying, "Cut back." It shows you *how* to cut back day by day, and systematically, and in a way that will allow you to feel comfortable and not deprived.

The mistake most people make when confronted with the need to change their behavioral patterns—in this case, the excessive consumption of foods that are killing them—is that they take the all-or-nothing approach. They say, okay, I'm not going to eat these things anymore, and then, when they find that their habits are too entrenched to abruptly break, they feel frustration, weakness, or a sense of failure. The second principle of the CARE program teaches you the key to successful detoxification through a gradual reduction of the animal products you are accustomed to eating. You will be able to eat reasonable amounts of the animal products you desire, in the healthiest way, offsetting their harmful effects through new behaviors you will be using, and at the same time you will be realizing your goal to CARE for your body by cleansing and rejuvenating it energetically.

Once again, please keep in mind that these new techniques you will be learning are guidelines, not edicts. I keep repeating this over and over whenever giving recommendations because people tend to view any digression from the guidelines as failure, which serves only to add undue pressure to realizing the goal at hand. Plus, I would rather overstress this idea than understress it. It simply is not realistic for me to try to address every possible variable, life circumstance, and personal choice of everyone in one book. So the guidelines serve as a pool of suggestions that can be drawn upon to satisfy each person's individual needs.

In the figure below, you will see that the area marked with an A is the largest, with B and C equal to each other but very much smaller. This is a way to illustrate the extent to which people practice certain habits. For example, if it were to show how often people exercise, the area marked A would represent the number of people who exercise at least sometimes. The

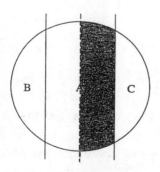

area marked B would represent the people who exercise every day, and the area marked C would represent those who never exercise.

Here, it is used to illustrate to what extent people eat animal products. The large Area A is the percentage of people who eat some form of animal product daily. Area B is the percentage of people who eat some animal products at every meal, and Area C is the percentage of those who never eat animal products.

Areas B and C have no varying degrees. You either eat animal products at every meal or you don't eat them at all. Area A however, can have a wide and varying range of amounts of animal products eaten. Now, in terms of reducing animal products sufficiently to promote cleanliness of the inner body, keep your lymph nodes from swelling, keep energy levels high, and optimize health, while preventing ill health, you want your level of consumption of animal products to be in the shaded part of Area A (to the right of the dashed line) that is closer to area C. Somewhere in there should be your goal. Obviously, the closer to Area C, the fewer animal products you are eating. The closer to the dashed line, the more animal products you're eating.

To achieve the goal of being in the shaded area next to Area C, there are three simple, general guidelines to strive for. I emphasize again that they are general guidelines. I will refer to flesh foods when talking about meat, chicken, fish, and eggs, and dairy products to indicate any milk product, including cheese, yogurt, sour cream, and so on.

1. Try to avoid eating flesh foods and/or dairy products for breakfast.

2. Try to have flesh foods no more than once a day. Try to have dairy products no more than once a day. (On occasion, you will have both more than once a day, but again, I am talking about direction. The direction you're going in is to strive for no more than once a day.)

3. On some kind of regular basis, there should be some days where neither flesh foods nor dairy products are eaten at all. This is exceedingly important. The body needs a break from having to expend energy on processing animal products. I know people who only eat animal products every other day. They do not feel deprived in any way and they experience phenomenal good health. One small exception for nonanimal-product days is the use of a little butter on potatoes or vegetables or when cooking something that requires butter. This small digression will not hurt anything. And by all means, use butter not margarine, which is nothing but plastic fat and has been associated with a significant increase in the risk of cancer.[232] At least, butter is real.

It is obvious that the more closely you adhere to and use these three guidelines, the more successful you will be in reducing your animal product consumption. One of the ways you can be more successful in implementing these tips is to understand as much as you can about why they are relevant. I have already given you ample reasons to cut back on animal products as you begin to CARE for your body. This is just one more understanding you will be able to incorporate into your lifestyle and use to your benefit for the rest of your life.

BENEFITS OF THE SECOND PRINCIPLE

These tips may appear to be too simplistic to have any major impact on supporting the lymph system and preventing disease, but just the opposite is true. If you practice them diligently and incorporate them into your lifestyle, you will contribute greatly to your goal of vibrant health.

We have already seen that elimination is an integral part of cleansing. It is the actual removal of waste matter through the bowels, the bladder, the lungs, and the skin, and because it cannot proceed without energy from the body, your dietary choices and your lifestyle will dramatically affect it. If most of the foods you eat are highly processed, full of chemicals, heavy, concentrated, high in fat and cholesterol, denatured, preserved, or irradiated, you can expect that elimination will not be smooth. Too much energy will be required by the body merely to break down these foods and neutralize their negative elements, and unless you are like the lion, who sleeps twenty hours a day, your body simply will not be able to thoroughly eliminate the waste products and toxins from the foods you are eating. Yes, it will eliminate somewhat, but not completely, and complete elimination is the key to a clean lymph system and the prevention of disease in general.

The idea in upgrading your diet is to gradually remove from your diet those foods that have been proven to be harmful. All I can tell you is that the fresher the food, the closer to nature, the better. You want to minimize your consumption of highly pro-cessed, chemicalized, packaged foods; coffee; soft drinks; refined sugar; and so on. You know the stuff that's not good for you. It's what we're always being told to "have in modera-tion." You will never hear an admonishment to eat fresh fruits and vegetables in moderation. Do the best you can in mini-mizing them. That's all. With periodic monodieting and reduc-ing animal products, you are way ahead of the game. You can get away with periodic indiscretions with no problem because your overall approach is so healthy.

World-renowned biochemist and researcher Dr. Paul Stitt has said, "The cure for cancer will not be found under the microscope, it's on the dinner plate."[233] The more foods that come from the plant kingdom, and the less that come from the animal kingdom, the less likely it is that cells will be driven crazy or any other disease will ever be part of your experience.

If you have decided that periodic monodieting and the grad-ual reduction of animal products make sense to you, and you are willing to apply the three CARE principles to your life, you will begin to make the health-supporting dietary choices so many others are making (and that you have perhaps been secretly yearning to know how to make), in a rational, systematic, and very enjoyable way. CARE gives you a comprehensive game plan for life, rather than a haphazard, hit-or-miss approach. You don't have to hope you will get results. From the moment you start, you will know you are getting them.

These principles will change forever the attitude you have toward your body, as you experience firsthand your own power to revitalize your physical body. You will be witnessing your ability to eliminate, by your own actions and behavior, the underlying causes of ill health that you thought were beyond your control. The result will be a higher level of health and energy than perhaps you ever thought possible! And most important, you will live with the knowledge and confidence that you can go through this life in vibrant health.

THIRTEEN

The Third Principle: The Mind Matters

If we are to be well and happy, not only the body, but the mind also must be peaceful and harmonious.

—Ernest Holmes,
The Science of Mind

It is well documented that in a climate of negativity, the ability to heal is greatly reduced—depressed people not only lower their immune response, for example, but even weaken their DNA's ability to repair itself.

—Deepak Chopra, M.D.,
Quantum Healing

Many of [the mind's] effects are achieved directly on the body's tissues without any awareness on our part. The body responds to the mind's messages whether conscious or unconscious.

—Bernie S. Siegel, M.D.,
Love, Medicine and Miracles

Your thoughts create your experience of your health, wealth and every detail of your world.

—Wayne Dyer, M.D.,
Real Magic

If you would perfect your body, guard your mind.

—James Allen,
As A Man Thinketh

What things soever you desire, when you pray, believe that you receive them, and you shall have them.

—Jesus

All that we are is the result of what we have thought.

—Buddha

The temptation was there to continue the list of quotations above and let seventy or eighty of them make up this chapter, so great is the amount of material that has been written over the years on the inextricable relationship between the mind and the body. The two parts of the mind that can be discussed are: that part which we know something about; and that part about which nothing is known. Studying the mind is like studying the cosmos itself.

What is actually known about the mind can be likened to a single grain of sand on a vast stretch of beach. Nevertheless, the tiny bit that we do know about is extraordinary and super-charged with power. And it is a power we can use! It is what Norman Cousins is referring to when he says, "The growth of the human mind is still high adventure, in many ways the highest adventure on earth."[234]

Have you ever heard statements like, "Attitude is everything," or "You are what you think you are," or "Your mind can make a heaven of hell or a hell of heaven"? Have you heard athletes refer to their "mental game" and the role it played in a win or loss? Indeed, one of the most renowned tennis instructors in the world told me that the game of tennis is 10 percent talent, 90 percent mental. In fact, you'll hear tennis players frequently say before a match, "If my mental game is there, I'll win." And after a loss, "My mental game just wasn't there."

You know the story of the little engine going up a steep hill, don't you? "I think I can, I think I can, I think I can," she says, and she does. And of course, the Master Teacher, Jesus, tried to teach us all this lesson when he said, over and over again in many different ways, "It is done unto you as you believe." What other possible meaning could this statement have but that the power of the mind, through right thinking, can bring into our experience absolutely anything we desire.

Volumes have been written on the power of the mind and its ability to strengthen us or weaken us, uplift us or bring us down, heal us or make us sick. And yet, although there is more than ample evidence that the mind, properly channeled, can be one of the most potent tools in the health and healing of the body, no other area of health care has been more minimized and neglected. It seems that when we cross from the seen to the unseen, all manner of biases come into play. As long as we're dealing with the physical world, the world that we can hear, see, or touch, we're comfortable. As soon as we move to that part of our existence that has no presence that we can relate to with our physical senses, the terra firma gets mighty shaky. There's an air of hocus-pocus, or cultism, or some other such nonsense attributed to the idea of the power of the mind to heal.

All you have to do to see that this is an area well worth your consideration is to read any of the books by Dr. Deepak Chopra, Dr. Wayne Dyer, Louise Hay, Dr. Bernie Siegel, or Ernest Holmes; you will learn about the many remarkable instances of people using their minds to send positive messages of love and healing to their bodies to overcome even catastrophic cases of disease.

THE MIND-BODY CONNECTION

In the physical world, it is well understood that there are natural laws that are simple and undeviating. If one plants the seed for a peach tree, a peach tree will grow. On the other hand, if the seed for a thistle bush is planted, there will be no peaches, only thistles. You may say that this is simple and obvious. But few understand that in the mental world, the law still holds true and is just as unyielding.

Your thoughts are like seeds in that thoughts become things, the same way seeds become plants. Good thoughts produce good things and negative thoughts produce negative things. Good thoughts will never produce negative results, and negative thoughts will never produce good results.

Although far too many medical scientists are quick to discount the role the mind plays in healing, favoring drugs instead, there is a wealth of scientific evidence that proves the astounding power of the mind to heal. In the area of psychiatry and psychology, there has been an explosion in mind-body research over the last decade. Dr. Martin Seligman, a professor at the University of Pennsylvania and author of *Learned Optimism,* has done research showing that pessimistic people have weaker "immune systems," are more prone to colds and flu, and have more major health problems after age fifty. Their bodies are less likely to fight off killer diseases such as cancer.

A colleague of Dr. Seligman's, Dr. Gregory Buchanon, also a researcher at the University of Pennsylvania, conducted tests on a group of subjects to determine if they were essentially pessimists or optimists. According to Dr. Buchanon, more of those who were identified as pessimists died within ten years. Those who ranked within the top 25 percent as the most negative had the highest death rate: 26 of 31 subjects died. By contrast, only 10 of the 31 who ranked as the most optimistic had died.[235]

THE PLACEBO EFFECT

Some of the most impressive and convincing evidence of the power of the mind to heal the body comes from what is referred to as the "placebo effect." In studies to determine the effectiveness of a drug, subjects afflicted with a certain malady are divided into two groups. One group receives the drugs to be tested, the other group receives a dummy pill or placebo, usually a coated sugar pill. Neither group knows which it is receiving, the real drug or the placebo. If the group receiving the real drug shows a marked improvement over the placebo group, the drug is deemed effective. But what has happened over and over again is that, for some people, the placebo turned out to be as effective as the drug. Not everyone responds this way, but generally 30 to 60 percent report relief of pain, even stabbing pain, from the placebo.[236]

Stated differently, being convinced of the potential effectiveness of a particular medicine or surgical procedure actually assists in making one well and improves one's chances of recovery. Conversely, feelings of skepticism and doubt in the same situation will bring about the exact opposite, less of a chance of recovery.[237] This phenomenon has been noted for centuries![238] At the beginning of the twentieth century Dr. William Osler enjoyed enormous fame as a physician and healer. He taught his students that his patients were frequently healed because of their faith in the treatment they received, not the treatment itself.[239]

One of the most celebrated cases in the history of the mind as healer of the body occurred early in the 1800s and involved Dr. Isaac Jennings. After twenty years of practicing medicine, Dr. Jennings became so disillusioned with drugging and bleeding his patients that he discontinued the treatments. To meet the demands of his patients for "medicines," he gave them an assortment of bread pills, a variety of powders made of wheat flour variously scented and colored, and vials of pure water of various hues. Much to his surprise, his patients made recoveries far in excess of what he saw when he administered drugs.

It was not long before Dr. Jennings's fame spread far and wide and his practice extended over a large territory, putting drugging doctors out of business. He continued substituting his innocent placebos for fifteen to twenty years before he revealed to his medical colleagues and to the community what he had been doing. Some of his colleagues were intrigued. Others were angry at him. Some of his patients said they didn't care what he gave them, because whatever it was it had healed them. Some were angry and called him an impostor and refused to continue to see him. The fact that the duration of their illnesses had been greatly shortened did not weigh in Dr. Jennings's favor. They paid for drugs and they wanted drugs. In spite of the puzzling, mixed reactions of his patients, Yale University conferred an honorary degree upon Dr. Jennings in recognition of his success.[240]

The reason placebos work is that the people taking them are convinced that they will help. They *think* the treatment will make them well, so it does! Placebos support the fact that positive beliefs enhance healing. Many present-day "authorities" doubt the scientific validity of the ability of the mind to heal the body, in spite of the fact that there exists a large body of scientific evidence that supports the argument that the mind has the power to heal the body. There are examples galore, all documented, of people healing themselves—sometimes of some very serious problems—all with their minds, their thoughts. They so strongly believed they were going to get well that they did! Take a look at Dr. Larry Dossey's *Healing Words,* a most fascinating and informative book (by a medical doctor) on the subject of the power of prayer to heal.

This awesome power resides in you right now. Nothing prevents you from using it on your own behalf other than your own thoughts. Whatever you want to call it, be it a positive mental attitude or the power of prayer, that power *will* respond to your thoughts, words, and beliefs. If you wish to make the determination with absolute certainty that you have tremendous influence over your health and well-being and know that it is so, you can! Indeed, you can just as easily think you are in charge as not.

Before giving you the tools to help you start to redirect your mind to think in a more positive light about the power you have over your own health, let's look at just a few of the more impressive examples of the placebo effect. Placebos have provided relief in cases of angina, arthritis, pain, hay fever, headaches, coughs, ulcers, hypertension, cancer, and heart disease.[241] Numerous studies of certain religious practices have shown a direct correlation between deeply held beliefs and the lessening of health problems.[242] One ten-year study on elderly people showed that those who actually thought of themselves and labeled themselves as old or elderly had significantly higher death rates over the course of the study than those who thought of themselves as middle-aged.[243]

The number of documented cases that prove the power of the mind to heal the body would easily fill this entire book. I will share two particularly striking illustrations, pertaining to the two biggest killers in North America—heart disease and cells gone crazy.

In the late 1950s and early 1960s, a new operation for the relief of angina became quite successful and popular. Angina is the medical term for pain, and it causes sudden and severe discomfort of the lower chest accompanied by a feeling of suffocation. If it is not dealt with, it is often a precursor of a more serious heart condition because it is a warning that blood flow to the heart is being restricted. Anyone who has experienced this excruciating pain does not cherish the idea of a repeat performance.

The operation, which has been largely replaced by what is referred to as a coronary bypass, involved opening the chest and ligating, or tying off, a certain artery in order to force more blood through other branches that were being obstructed. The operation brought a marked relief of pain in 70 percent of patients. In a controlled study, randomly selected patients who were to receive this operation were anesthetized and an incision in the chest was made in the appropriate area, and that was all that was done. There was no tying off of the arteries or anything else. The incision was closed up and the patients were told it was a successful operation. These individuals, believing they'd had the operation, experienced a 70 percent improvement in relief of their pain, precisely the same degree of relief as those who actually had their arteries tied off![244] Now, that's impressive stuff.

The second illustration of the power of the mind to heal the body is as startling as anything I have ever come across. This case pertains to a profoundly sick gentleman who, among other health problems, had large cancerous tumors all over his body. All standard treatments had been tried and abandoned, and he was not expected to survive another month. At the time, there was a widely touted cancer "cure" called Krebiozen. The man heard about it and felt it would help him and begged for it to be administered to him. His condition was so bad that he must have thought there would be no harm by trying it; after all, he was already so close to death.

Two days after the first injection, the man's tumors had shrunk to one-half their original size. He was given injections three times a week and was discharged from the hospital in ten days. He enjoyed two months of practically perfect health, but as fate would have it, he received some conflicting reports on Krebiozen. He immediately relapsed to his preterminal state. The tumors returned. His physicians told him to disregard what he'd read because they were going to give him a new "double-strength, superrefined batch of Krebiozen." He perked up with a very strong anticipation of cure, but this time was injected with distilled water. Nevertheless, the tumors once again melted away and he was again symptom-free for two more months! He then had occasion to read the final American Medical Association report that Krebiozen had been shown to be worthless. He died two days later.[245]

So powerful is the mind in creating whatever reality it is convinced of that up to 50 percent of subjects in some studies actually exhibit side effects from the placebos.[246] In one astonishing case involving the testing of an antihistamine, the subjects receiving the placebos experienced more side effects than those who received the medication![247] Results of recent studies show the placebo effect to be twice as powerful as previously thought,[248] and most powerful when a trusted physician enthusiastically offers a patient a new therapy.[249]

Given that there are people who accept suggestion from authority figures so strongly that they view the suggestion as reality and actually cause the expected result to occur, it should be a punishable crime for anyone in a position of authority to tell a patient that he or she is going to die or has but a short time left before dying. Even if there is a minuscule chance that a person would survive, it is ignorance and arrogance of the highest order for anyone to tell another person when he or she is going to die. That's God's decision. And only God knows how many people have been ushered to an early grave because they had the idea planted in their minds that their time was up. I wonder if there is *anyone* who hasn't heard of someone living far beyond the time they were told they would die.

Medical doctors have notoriously discounted the idea that the mind can heal the body. The American Medical Association queried their members in 1990 and found that only 10 percent believed in the mind-body connection.[250] Nevertheless, wouldn't the decent thing be to tell a patient about those instances where other patients conquered the disease and survived or beat the odds? I cannot think of one woman I know who had a mastectomy who was not told her choice was either a mastectomy or death. It's just not right. The death-sentence approach in our health-care system is one that sorely needs to be changed.

GUIDELINES TO POSITIVE THINKING

After what you've read, you could easily be thinking that the mind might be the most powerful tool of all in your quest to achieve vibrant health. And who's to say you would not be right? The task for many of us, however, is to figure out how to retrain ourselves to think in such a way as to take full advantage of the potential that resides in the mind, the same way a mighty oak tree resides in a single acorn. Under the right circumstances, that acorn will become the oak tree. And under the right circumstances, the extraordinary and dynamic source of power that is the mind will unleash its gifts. It waits patiently for your direction.

If your commitment to health is such that you will be periodically monodieting and gradually reducing your consumption of animal products, the addition of your knowing, really knowing, that your efforts will prevent you from ever becoming sick creates a winning combination that vastly improves your chances of success. But trying to turn around a lifetime of negative thinking, or thinking that is not supportive to your goals, can be a challenge. Like other habits that have become fixed or routine, the way to change them is to crowd them out with other, more favorable ones.

There is no question that you can accomplish this. You are in charge of how you think, and at any moment you have the choice to change your thoughts in any direction you wish. The mind is enormously receptive to your directives. It doesn't matter how long you have been thinking negatively. You can instantly turn it around by positive thoughts that will override negative ones right away. It's like turning on a light in a dark room. No matter how long the room has been dark, the moment you switch on the light, the darkness is removed.

In all likelihood there are hundreds of tools or guidelines you could use to assist you in training the mind to think about your daily life in a more positive way. Consider the following three that I and thousands of others have used with enormous success, and that you can use specifically to help in your quest to live a pain-free, disease-free life:

1. Ask better questions.
2. State your best case to the universe.
3. Acknowledge and accept your many "I's."

ASK BETTER QUESTIONS

This is a tool that can bring about remarkable, almost miraculous results, is as easy as anything could ever be, and is interesting and fun to use. I first learned about the power of questions from Anthony Robbins, author of the best-sellers *Unlimited Power* and *Awaken the Giant Within.* I have been friends with Tony for nearly twenty years, and he is one of the most consistently positive people I have ever known.

You may not even be aware of it, but you are constantly asking yourself questions either silently or out loud, and your brain is constantly supplying answers. "Ask and you shall receive." Most people have heard this phrase from the Bible. When you ask for something from the brain, it snaps right to attention and answers. It's just like a computer that contains millions of pieces of information. You punch in a question and up pops the answer on the screen. Whatever you ask of yourself, good or bad, receives an answer. So if you ask, "Why can't I ever lose weight?" your brain tells you why you can't. "Well, you eat too much, you don't try hard enough, you're not serious, you don't exercise enough, you were born that way."

Your brain will come up with an answer. So questions have the power to create positiveness or negativeness in your life. But what if you asked instead, "How can I lose weight and enjoy myself while I'm doing it?" Wouldn't you rather have an answer to that question?

Have you asked any of these?

"Why can't I ever get ahead?"
"Why does this always happen to me?"
"Why does so and so always treat me so badly?"
"Why am I so fat?"
"Why am I always suffering from one thing or another?"

If you ask why you can't do something, your brain will tell you why and you compound your unwanted situation. The secret of turning this around is to ask better questions! You can make a major positive change in your life starting right now with the right questions. It has a lot to do with what you choose to focus on. You see, whatever you focus on, you get! The decision is yours and no one else's. You can focus on what's good in your life or what's not. It's totally up to you.

If you watch the news on television and hear a story about some heinous crime, and later hear a story about a group that takes children with balloons to visit a retirement home just to bring some joy and light into the lives of the folks who live there, on which story would you focus? There are people who focus on all the pain and suffering in the world, and there are those who choose to see the beauty and goodness that exists in the world. You always have a choice to focus on either the positive or the negative in your life.

If you focus on how things just don't seem to work out, they won't! But guess what? The opposite is also true. Focus on how things *will* work out and they will. Remember: "It is done unto you as you believe."

The only difference between you and people you admire greatly for what they have achieved and the positive feelings they always seem to project is what you have chosen to focus on and what questions you ask of yourself. You can be sure that people like Anthony Robbins, and the people you admire most, are not asking themselves negative, disempowering questions. They're the ones asking questions like, "How can I turn this around and benefit from it?" instead of "Why does this always happen to me?" They are asking the kinds of questions that constantly spur them on to more and more achievements.

If you want things to work out in terms of your health goals, you must decide on what you're going to focus and what questions you're going to ask yourself. The right question can change your focus and that can change your life. Ever hear the story of the man who constantly lamented not having any shoes until he met another man without any feet? His focus changed in a hurry.

This all may sound so simple, even silly, but it makes such a massive difference, it would be a tragedy to have this powerful tool right in front of you and not take advantage of it.

As you pursue your goal to live happily, healthfully, and disease-free, always be asking yourself positive, uplifting questions:

"How can I support myself today to be healthier?"
"What can I do to specifically assist my lymph system's effort to remove toxins and waste from my body?"
"What can I do to make exercise more interesting and enjoyable?"
"What will I do with all of the newfound energy I'm going to have?"
"What did I do to be so blessed to find this information?"

Regularly ask yourself positive questions; this will create a positive atmosphere around you, and good things will happen as a result. And before you ask a question like, "Gee, do you think this can really work?" ask instead, "How can I *make* this work?"

Here's something you can start doing tomorrow morning that will progressively make you stronger and stronger, and more positive about CAREing for your body. Before you even get out of bed, just take a few moments each morning to start the day off with a couple of positive questions.

Have you ever awakened in the morning with the question on your lips, "Why do I have to go to work today?" or some other negative-based question? Not a very good way to start the day.

What if you woke up and said, "What can I do today to make it a more joyous day?"

If you will think of a general group of positive questions to ask yourself every morning, you will energize your entire life. Here's a sampling, but please add your own as well:

"What am I happiest about in my life?"
"What are the things I have to be grateful for?"
"Who are my friends?"
"Who loves me?"
"What have I accomplished that I'm deeply proud of?"

Before leaping out of bed and tackling the tasks of the day, lie there and ask yourself positive questions and briefly answer them to yourself. It will take three to five minutes to ask and answer these questions.

What if you started every day like that? You might begin to buzz with positive energy! If this became a habit in your life every morning, just like brushing your teeth, over time, merely waking up would automatically put you into a positive state. This is how the mind can be retrained to think in a way that is more supportive of the healthy lifestyle you desire. One last question to ponder: "Isn't it great that you are so open to making these positive changes to improve your life, and these tools are now available to help you?"

STATE YOUR BEST CASE TO THE UNIVERSE

Have you ever been in someone's home or office and seen either on the wall, desk, or table a plaque with some kind of inspirational or uplifting quotation or saying? Why do you think they are displayed in such prominent places? Do you have these kinds of inspirational messages around your home or office? If so, why? The answer couldn't be more obvious. They are designed to inspire the reader, to remind the reader of all the good and positive things that can exist. When you read a message of love or happiness or success or some other positive aspect of life, for those few moments while you are reading it, don't you feel good? If it's particularly applicable to something that is happening to you at the time, don't you kind of purse your lips a little, nod in recognition, and think, "Of course, of course"? It's as though the message was written just for you.

The written word can be, and is, enormously powerful. "The pen is mightier than the sword" is a wise saying that illustrates the point. Words written on a page can make you weep or make you laugh, make you sad or make you happy, make you feel anger or make you feel compassion. When you read something, it is imprinted in your mind's eye. Have you ever heard the name of a person or place or object of some kind and not been able to pronounce it properly until you saw it written down?

The power inherent in writing something down is the very reason so many people write affirmations on a regular basis. Say, for example, someone is desperately trying to find a job that is more rewarding both financially and professionally. He or she may write the affirmation: "I know that the position I am looking for that is perfect for me will present itself soon." It may be written one time, ten times, fifty times or a hundred times every day. The affirmation becomes a permanent part of the person's consciousness, a way of thinking that leaves no room for anything but what is desired. That is why so many people believe in writing goals down on paper. Seminars are held all over the country on goal setting to show people exactly how to use it to attract what they desire. Invariably these seminars involve the writing down on paper what they wish to come into their lives.

Other people will write a word on a piece of paper every morning with the idea of concentrating on that one word all day, such as "health," "love," "peace," "compassion," "forgiveness," "success," "joy," "concentration" or any number of different possibilities. The next day another word is written down, and it is the focus of attention for the day.

There are many tools such as these to use the written word not only to attract what you want, but also to train your mind to focus in a positive rather than negative way. One approach I have used for years that works well with the first tool of asking better questions is stating something as fact rather than asking about it. This can be done with one, two, three, four, or however many statements you wish. Write neatly on a piece of paper statements of fact as you wish them to be. For example:

- My body is becoming cleaner, stronger, and healthier every day.
- My lymph system is working at optimum efficiency, preventing cells from ever being driven crazy.
- My lymph nodes are clean and they are going to stay that way.
- I am open and receptive to the vast number of possibilities available to me.
- I enjoy the work I have chosen to perform and it is important.
- Outer circumstances cannot disturb my sense of well-being. I am in charge of my happiness.
- My life is supercharged with all the energy I need to be happy and well.

I have many of these statements posted all around my home. I would like to share with you one that I saw many years ago and I have been reading to myself every day, sometimes several times a day, ever since. It sits on my desk where I write and I always read it before I begin my writing day:

> I go forth as an empowered and an empowering person. I come from strength, and I bring strength into all that I do. I call upon inner wisdom and love to guide me in the right use of my time and talents, all to bring a greater good to life.

Remember, there can be as many or as few of these statements as you like on any subject whatsoever. You then put the piece of paper with the most empowering statements you can think of in some conspicuous place where you will be sure to see it during the day. On your desk, on the refrigerator, on the dashboard of your car, anywhere. You then make a commitment to read these insights at least once a day. This can be at any time during the day that you feel is most convenient, upon awakening in the morning, before going to sleep at night, at lunchtime. I'm not talking about a huge expenditure of time. It takes less time to read these statements than to see what's on television tonight. When you read the statements, don't just read them mechanically, say them to yourself with feeling and conviction. *Mean it!*

Now, you may be asking, if it's being suggested to read them just once a day, why do they have to be in a conspicuous place? If you are asking that question, then you are really paying attention, so thank you. This is the reason I keep these statements conspicuously placed: Being a writer, I spend considerable time at my desk. My statements are within easy grasp. As it happens, as I pause to ponder something pertaining to my work, I can see the statements sitting there. This has two benefits. First, it's so easy to read one or two of the statements, which immediately refocuses my thoughts and gives me an energy boost, making sure my thoughts remain positive and high-minded. Second, after you have made the daily reading of your statements a habit and you have been doing it for several weeks or months, just seeing the piece of paper with the statements on it instantly has the same effect as reading one or more of them.

You know what's on the list. So every time you look at it, you are, in effect, keeping your mind on track—the positive track. You can add or delete statements at any time, and to be sure, feel free to read them as many times a day as you wish. The minimum is one time, but you can't read them too often. Please don't underestimate this approach. It is a powerful tool as you will quickly find out.

ACKNOWLEDGE AND ACCEPT YOUR MANY "I'S"

Have you ever made comments similar to these:

"I don't know what came over me. That's just not like me at all."
"I had a real battle with myself."
"I can't make up my mind. I keep going back and forth."
"If I did that, I'd never forgive myself."
"One moment I want to do one thing, the next moment I want to do the opposite."

Do these statements sound at all familiar? It is probably a safe bet to say that at one time or another we have all had thoughts like these. It's as though there is more than one person living in our bodies all with their own likes and dislikes, wants and needs, and all vying to be heard and be in charge. The idea may sound a bit odd to you, but is a point of view held by quite a few people around the world and one which was written about extensively by one of the world's most intriguing philosophers, George Gurdjieff. His writings and writings about him have been the object of study and discussion by large numbers of people all around the world.

One of the central themes of Gurdjieff's philosophy was that we all have many "I's" but that we don't realize it. Because we have one body and one name, we think we are one. But we are many. We may have dozens, perhaps hundreds, of lesser I's all wanting to be heard.

What exactly do I mean when I say I's? The I's refer to the different parts of you that want different things at different times. For example, "I want to buckle down and get on a good diet and lose some weight." Now, when these words are spoken, they're meant! But at another time of day, that particular I's resolve is weakened and a different I says, "I want to enjoy myself and eat whatever I like." These two I's are each trying to get an upper hand over the other. "That does it. I'm going to start exercising a half hour at least four times a week. I'm going to get in shape."

You say it with absolute conviction. Then,

"I have so much to think about, I'm going to start exercising first thing next month."
"I want to clean out the garage."
"I want to kick back, read a novel, and have some chocolate."
"I'm going to put in some extra hours at work and really solidify my position there."
"I can't wait to get home and just forget about work."
"I want to read a good book."
"I want to go to the movies."
"I'm going to have a really healthy lunch today."
"I want a burger and fries."
"I want to do more with the children on the weekend."
"I just want to take it easy and do nothing this weekend."

"I want to go out tonight."
"I want to stay home."

And on and on and on for practically every situation in life. The fact is, each and every one of these statements is real! When they are spoken, the I that is in charge is speaking for the whole, even though many other I's may disagree but do not have the floor at that moment. Think of fictional Jane Doe going through a day: Each of her separate I's is able to call itself Jane, is able to act in her name, agree or disagree in her name, make decisions or promises in her name with which another I in Jane will have to cope. This explains why people so often make decisions that are frequently not carried out. One I makes the decision, another I ignores it. It's as though someone writes a check in your name and then you have to make good on it.

Understanding this aspect of your life can be very freeing. You can start to recognize certain I's and become familiar with them. Once you know which ones are there and how they operate, you can start to bring them in line with the I's that are more aligned with your quest for vibrant health. You know that there are I's in you that absolutely want to eat properly and exercise regularly. And there are other I's in you that don't. Just having that understanding is a breakthrough.

Each I, whether a strong, positive one or a weak, negative one, wants to have its way whenever it can. It wants to do what it is accustomed to doing and does not want to change or allow any other I to take precedence.

This creates a lot of turmoil in people who are not aware of the many I's and don't know what's causing them so much indecision and anguish. But when you know what's going on, you can observe the different I's and even say out loud to the ones you know don't care about your well-being, "So, you're back. Here to try and influence me to disregard my health, are you?" Of course, this confrontation with the I is to be done in private. If you do it in front of people, they may start to chase you with a big butterfly net. Standing around shaking your finger at yourself, admonishing yourself to go away and leave yourself alone could attract the wrong kind of attention. But observing the different I's that come up in a day and confronting them can be very interesting. And only when you recognize that they're there can you begin to take charge of them and create some order.

Knowing this theory of the many I's, the next time you say something like, "I can't believe I ate those doughnuts. I don't know what I was thinking. I'm trying to cleanse and rejuvenate my body!," you will know that there are two different I's at work. One wanting to CARE for itself, the other hell-bent on momentary pleasure, no matter how destructive. The more you observe this phenomenon, the more familiar you will become with your own diverse makeup, and the more likely you will be able to give dominance to the I's that support your health goals and maintain a positive direction in your life.

You can also stop browbeating yourself or feeling guilty about one thing or another you did or wish you didn't do, or didn't do and wish you did. Just know that at some times different I's are stronger than at other times and forgive yourself your human frailty. Better to work at strengthening your positive I's than bemoaning the action of your negative ones.

The idea of many I's all vying for control can be likened to a house being built by a group of workers with no supervisor in charge. The workers have not been instructed as to their specific duties, so each, feeling he knows best what to do, tries his hand at being in charge. But others feel they could handle the situation better and disagreements erupt.

The building of the house is not progressing in an orderly fashion. Instead, there is chaos. The only chance is for the supervisor to show up and organize everyone and assign the right job to the right person so the entire crew is working as a team. When it comes to your many I's, the "supervisor" in this case would be your strong, positive, health-seeking I, the one that is committed to keeping you on track and seeking out the most supportive conditions in your life. The only way to make this I stronger and more capable of governing the other I's is to habitually perform certain practices that will strengthen it and give it power and confidence. There is an I in you that wants to believe, that *does* believe, that you have the information, the tools, and the ability to live a vibrantly healthy life free of pain and disease.

There is also the I that doesn't, so anything you can do to strengthen the positive I and silence the negative I is going to weigh heavily in your success. By recognizing that you have these different I's, and consciously asking better questions so your strong I's will answer, and stating your intentions to the universe, you are taking a huge step in strengthening the strong, positive, health-seeking I that *knows* you will never become sick, so that it is the one that predominates in your life.

EMOTIONS AND SELF-HEALING

There is one last issue I must address as regards cells being driven crazy, either preventing it or beating it. Although this is an area of immense importance, it somehow has received scant attention. As indicated earlier, there are many variables that contribute to cells being driven crazy. I have focused primarily on the effects of diet on health both because I am certain that is the main risk factor, and because diet happens to be my area of expertise.

Scholars and researchers have shown that repressed, un-vented anger, coupled with a lack of self-love, has been a major contributor in many cases of all kinds of disease. Although this is not my area of expertise, it would be remiss of me if I did not bring it to your attention and encourage you to take a close, hard look at this area of your life. To help you do so, I would like to introduce you to the work of a most remarkable woman.

Louise L. Hay is an internationally respected author and

lecturer. I have the very good fortune of having a personal relationship with Ms. Hay and I can tell you without hesitation that she is one of the most genuinely loving, compassionate, and concerned people I have ever met. Merely being in the same room with her lifts your spirits and fills you with good feelings.

Ms. Hay was diagnosed with incurable, terminal cancer. Even if she were to submit to incredibly extensive surgery, her chance of survival, she was told, was nil. She rejected the medical approach entirely, and instead decided to focus on why she had such negative feelings about herself. She scrutinized the abuses she had endured both as a child and as an adult and realized the full extent to which these unresolved issues had been fermenting within her, culminating in cancer. She simultaneously detoxified her body with a cleansing diet.

In one of the most remarkable instances of self-healing I have ever heard of, Louise Hay totally healed herself! Only six months after diagnosis, her doctors told her there was not even a trace of cancer. This was many years ago and she is still cancer-free.

Ms. Hay's many books and tapes are available to you. I suggest that you take a look at *You Can Heal Your Life,* which has been read by millions worldwide. I know people whose lives have been changed merely by reading this book. You can be one of them.

THE BENEFITS OF THE THREE CARE PRINCIPLES

The stronger you become, the more you will want to use the three principles of CARE I have laid out. The frequency with which you use them depends entirely on your level of motivation. How quickly do you want to start to cleanse and strengthen your lymph system, which in turn protects you against becoming sick? How truly committed are you to experiencing a long life dominated by high spirits, vitality, and health, rather than aches, pains, and illness?

These are the kinds of questions we are all grappling with. At night when you lay your head on your pillow and you are alone with your thoughts in the dark, these are issues that can loom large. By using the three CARE principles, with an attitude of knowing that they will work and that ill health will never be a part of your life, you will be able to live out your life in health, confident that you are the one in control of your destiny.

FOURTEEN

You Have a Choice

In an article in the *New York Times,* Dr. Yitzhak Koch states that "The breast is a unique gland, an underestimated gland. Its activity is much more complex than people had thought."[251] And I would like to add to that, that a woman's breasts are exactly where they belong. So is a man's prostate gland, and every other part of the body that God put there. They do not have to be removed and they do not have to be mutilated. You can prevent cells from ever being driven crazy in your body; there is no doubt whatsoever about it. It is a daunting challenge, I know, especially in light of the "experts," who are supposed to know how, declaring that they don't.

What I have offered in this book is one way to prevent this phenomenon from occurring, and the years of pain, ill health, and anguish that precede it. There may be other ways, to be sure, and if there are, I am hopeful that they will be discovered and offered to people everywhere so that the suffering can end. Preventing cells from being driven crazy is not something that is accomplished by taking a onetime action that achieves the goal. It certainly would be lovely if there were a pill or a shot or some other "magic bullet" that would do the job and remove the need for ongoing diligence, but there isn't, and that's that.

If you have a doorway in your home that is too low and you bump your forehead every time you go through it, all you have to do to prevent that from happening is to have the doorway raised and that's the end of the problem. You don't have to think about it anymore. When it comes to the prevention of disease, it's not that simple. It's not one action that you perform. It's the way you choose to live your life. You can live in a manner that opens the way for pain and disease to develop, or you can live in a manner that produces vibrant health. To prevent disease, to really, truly prevent it, an ongoing effort is called for.

I may be accused of being naïve in thinking that by cleansing the lymph system, cutting back on animal products, exercising, and maintaining a positive attitude, something as seemingly complex and baffling as what we refer to as cancer can be prevented when medicine's greatest minds have not yet been able to get a handle on it. But my questions to you are these: What if I'm right? What if the approach suggested in this book will do the job? If it works, does it matter one way or the other that I'm not a medical doctor and that the approach is straightforward, uncomplicated, and not dependent upon expensive diagnostic procedures and invasive treatment?

I'm not saying that this book will end this particular disease, but I can tell you it will definitely prevent it for a lot of people and perhaps you are one of them. What do you have to lose by trying what I'm suggesting? Even if I'm wrong, what possible harm could there be in cleaning your inner body so it operates more efficiently, reducing your intake of the foods that every health professional recommends you should eat less of, exercising regularly, and keeping a positive mental attitude? You sure as the dickens will never see any of those things on a death certificate.

What else are you being offered? Remember, the experts

don't know how to prevent cancer, and only 5 percent of research money goes toward prevention. If you sit around and wait for some magic bullet, you might find yourself under the knife. That *must* be avoided. To do that, you must think prevention, prevention, prevention. If someone offers you something to prevent illness that makes more sense to you than what you have read here, then do it! By all means. But don't do nothing!

If you wait for early detection as it is being suggested to you, you have the disease. I guarantee, if you were to hear the words "I'm sorry, you have cancer," you would try anything to avoid losing a breast or your prostate gland and undergoing chemotherapy. Don't wait! The time is now and prevention is the key.

Devra Lee Davis is a specialist in public health policy and a scholar in residence at the National Research Council of the National Academy of Sciences, a prestigious position she has held since 1989. She has compiled one of the few systematic comparisons of current changes in deaths from cancer. With one out of three people a cancer victim in this country, we are all pained by the abysmal failure of the highly publicized and costly "war on cancer." Ms. Davis is fully aware of this situation as well, and when it comes to demanding change, she's not shy!

She rightly points out that the National Cancer Institute's 1982 goal of reducing cancer deaths by 50 percent by the end of the twentieth century looks ludicrous today. The mortality rate is actually higher than it was when the "war on cancer" began more than twenty years ago. Referring to the need to investigate further lifestyle changes such as diet and exercise and environmental causes, she states that, "The United States is not putting enough money into research on cancer prevention!"[252] She offers a plausible reason, too: "When you treat cancer, profits are made through drugs and surgery. But when cancer is prevented, nobody makes any money."[253] Ouch!

As you might well imagine, her public position has not exactly endeared her to the old boy network of the cancer establishment. Fortunately, standing outside the old boy network are progressive and enlightened physicians such as Dr. Edmund Sonnenblick, chairman of cardiology at Albert Einstein College of Medicine in New York. In Dr. Sonnenblick's words: "The public wants drama, but prevention is more important. The major thrust has to be prevention."[254]

At the end of the article on Ms. Davis in the *New York Times,* she ponders where the constituency for prevention is, and how hard building that constituency will be. It may be idealistic of me, or perhaps it's just positive thinking with a dash of wishful thinking thrown in, but in my opinion it's you who are that constituency. In taking this step to eliminate the causes of disease by CAREing for your body, you thereby distance yourself from the disease establishment and those who "don't know." You become a vital part of the real "health care" system—that network of health-conscious people who have taken charge of their lives and their health and are living the vibrant and vital life that our creator intended us to live.

Congratulations, and may God bless your every breath and step.

ENDNOTES

a. "Key Statistics." *World Health Organization*, World Health Organization, 3 Feb. 2012, www.who.int/cancer/resources/keyfacts/en/#:~:text=In%202008 %2C%207.6%20million%20people,and%20middle%2Dincome%2Dcoun tries.
b. "Cancer." *World Health Organization*, World Health Organization, 12 Sept. 2018, www.who.int/news-room/fact-sheets/detail/cancer.
c. Sandoiu, Ana. "Yo-Yo Dieting May Increase Risk of Heart Disease Death." *Medical News Today*, MediLexicon International, 15 Nov. 2016, www. medicalnewstoday.com/articles/314136.
1. "Activists Back More Money to Fight Cancer," *Washington Post,* Sept. 27, 1998.
2. Passwater, Richard A., Ph.D., *Cancer Prevention and Nutritional Therapies,* Keats, New Canaan, CT, 1993.
3. American Cancer Society, *Cancer Facts and Figures.*
4. Ibid.
5. Bailor, John, et al., "Cancer: Are We Losing the War?" *New England Journal of Medicine,* Vol. 314, May 8, 1986.
6. Ellerbee, Linda, "The Other Epidemic—What Every Woman Needs to Know About Breast Cancer," ABC-TV, Sept. 14, 1993; "Fighting Cancer—Are We Doing Enough?" CNN-Newsmaker, Sunday, July 7, 1991.
7. "Cancer War Has Stalled," *New York Times,* Oct. 30, 1994.

8. Cragg, Juli, "No Fault of Their Own," *Sarasota Herald-Tribune,* Dec. 5, 1993.
9. McDougall, John, M.D., *McDougall's Medicine: A Challenging Second Opinion,* New Century, Piscataway, NJ, 1985.
10. Ibid.
11. Rechweg, Hans, M.D., *Homitoxicology,* Nemaco Publishing, Albuquerque, NM, 1980.
12. Shelton, Herbert M., *Natural Hygiene: Man's Pristine Way of Life,* Dr. Shelton's Health School, TX, 1968.
13. Solomon, Neil, M.D., "Fever Still a Mystery," *Los Angeles Times,* Dec. 14, 1979.
14. Donohue, Paul, M.D., "Fever's Protective Role a Hot Topic," *Sarasota Herald-Tribune,* Aug. 9, 1999.
15. Seely, Rod R., Ph.D., Stephens, Trent D., Ph.D., Tate, Phillip, D.A., *Anatomy & Physiology*, Mosby, St. Louis, 1992.
16. "Breast Cancer—Speaking Out," PBS-TV, Oct. 13, 1993.
17. Sardi, P., "Winning Over the Public: The Battle Between Pharmaceutical and Nutritional Supplements," *Townsend Letter for Doctors,* July 1996, pp. 74–79.
18. Buchwald, Art, "Pill-Pushing for Fun and Profit," *Los Angeles Times,* Oct. 6, 1991.
19. "Rash of New Drugs Shot in Arm for Prescription Sales," Associated Press, Aug. 31, 1998.
[*Notes 20–34 were deleted in the previous edition.*]
35. Walker, N.W., M.D., *Become Younger,* Norwalk Press, Phoenix, 1979.
36. Guyton, A.C., M.D., *Medical Physiology,* W.B. Saunders, New York, 1962.
37. Shils, M., Olson, J., and Shike, M., eds., *Modern Nutrition in Health and Disease,* 8th ed., Lea & Febiger, Baltimore, 1994, p. 626.
38. Seely, Rod R., Ph.D., Stephens, Trent D., Ph.D., Tate, Phillip, D.A., *Anatomy & Physiology*, Mosby, St. Louis, 1992.
39. "Tonsils Bargain," *London Observer,* Feb. 21, 1988.
40. "The Breast Care Test." PBS-TV, Oct. 18, 1993.
41. Seely, Rod R., Ph.D., Stephens, Trent D., Ph.D., Tate, Phillip, D.A., *Anatomy & Physiology*, Mosby, St. Louis, 1992.
42. Foldi, M., *Lymphology,* Charles C Thomas, Springfield, 1969; Kleinsmith, L.J., and Rich, U.M., *Principles of Cell and Molecular Biology,* Harper-Collins, New York, 1995.
43. Waldman, Hilary, "Breast Cancer: Lymph Node Removal Re-examined," *Sarasota Herald-Tribune,* Sept. 11, 1996.
44. Janofsky, Michael, "Results of Biopsy Show Simpson to Be Cancer-Free, Doctor Says," *New York Times*, Aug. 16, 1994.
45. "Workers Told of Risks in Handling Cancer Drugs," *Los Angeles Times,* Sept. 13, 1983.

46. Friend, Tim, "Lymphoma's Progression Was Swift," *USA Today,* May 20, 1994; Altman, Lawrence K., "Doctors Told Mrs. Onassis There Was Nothing More They Could Do," *New York Times,* May 20, 1994.

47. Ibid.

48. Altman, Lawrence K., M.D., "Lymphomas Are on the Rise in U.S., and No One Knows Why," *New York Times,* May 24, 1994.

49. "Drop in Smoking Leads to Decline in Cancer Risks," Associated Press, April 21, 1999.

50. CNN Health Week, March 14, 1992; "No Breast, No Cancer," *Maury Povich Show,* June 18, 1992; "Pre-ventive Mastectomy, Part I & Part II," *Health Talk,* March 10 and 11, 1993; "Siblings Opt for Preventive Mastectomies," All Things Considered (National Public Radio), Aug. 8, 1993; Angier, Natalie, "Vexing Pursuit of Breast Cancer Gene," *New York Times,* July 12, 1994.

51. "The Breast Care Test," PBS-TV, Oct. 18, 1993.

52. Quillin, Patrick, M.D., *Beating Cancer with Nutrition,* NTP Press, Tulsa, OK, 1994.

53. Ellerbee, Linda, "The Other Epidemic—What Every Woman Needs to Know About Breast Cancer," ABC-TV, Sept. 14, 1993.

54. Stephen, Beverly, "Her Most Serious Medical Problem," *Los Angeles Times,* Dec. 5, 1982.

55. Ellerbee, Linda, "The Other Epidemic—What Every Woman Needs to Know About Breast Cancer," ABC-TV, Sept. 14, 1993.

56. Ellerbee, Linda, "The Other Epidemic—What Every Woman Needs to Know About Breast Cancer," ABC-TV, Sept. 14, 1993; "Fighting Cancer—Are We Doing Enough?" CNN Newsmaker, Sunday, July 7, 1991; "How Common Is Breast Cancer?: Breast Cancer Statistics." *American Cancer Society*, 8 Jan. 2020, www.cancer.org/cancer/breast-cancer/about/how-common-is-breast-cancer.html.

57. "Conflicting Advice in Breast Cancer," ABC *Night-line,* March 19, 1993.

58. *New England Journal of Medicine,* Oct. 24, 1985.

59. "Funds Urged for Breast Cancer Study," *The Associated Press*, Oct. 28, 1993.

60. Ellerbee, Linda, "The Other Epidemic—What Every Woman Needs to Know About Breast Cancer," ABC-TV, Sept. 14, 1993.

61. "The Breast Care Test," PBS-TV, Oct. 18, 1993.

62. Kolata, Gina, "Weighing Spending on Breast Cancer Research," *New York Times,* Oct. 20, 1993.

63. "Conflicting Advice in Breast Cancer," ABC *Night-line,* March 19, 1993.

64. Raloff, Janet, "EcoCancers," *Science News*, Vol. 144, No. 1, July 3, 1993.

65. "Conflicting Advice in Breast Cancer," ABC *Nightline,* March 19, 1993.

66. "The Breast Care Test," PBS-TV, Oct. 18, 1993.

67. Kolata, Gina, "Mammograms Before 50? A Hung Jury," *New York Times,* Nov. 24, 1993.
68. "Fighting Cancer—Are We Doing Enough?" CNN Newsmaker, Sunday, July 7, 1991.
69. Kolata, Gina, "Avoiding Mammogram Guidelines," *New York Times,* Dec. 5, 1993.
70. NBC *Nightly News,* Oct. 3, 1994.
71. Ibid.
72. "The Breast Care Test," PBS-TV, Oct. 18, 1993.
73. "It Could Happen to You," *ABC News—20/20,* Aug. 27, 1993.
74. Angier, Natalie, "Vexing Pursuit of Breast Cancer Gene," *New York Times,* July 12, 1994.
75. Angier, Natalie, "Move Abroad Can Change Breast Cancer Risk," *New York Times,* Aug. 2, 1995.
76. McDougall, John, M.D., *McDougall's Medicine: A Challenging Second Opinion,* New Century, Piscataway, NJ, 1985.
77. Elizabeth Berg, author of *Talk Before Sleep*, on the *Oprah Winfrey Show,* Aug. 1, 1994.
78. "Fighting Cancer—Are We Doing Enough?" CNN-Newsmaker, Sunday, July 7, 1991.
79. "Breast Cancer Defenses Sought," Associated Press (*Sarasota Herald-Tribune),* Dec. 15, 1993.
80. "The Breast Care Test," PBS-TV, Oct. 18, 1993.
81. "Conflicting Advice in Breast Cancer," ABC *Night-line,* March 19, 1993.
82. Kolata, Gina, "Mammograms Before 50? A Hung Jury," *New York Times,* Nov. 24, 1993.
83. Kolata, Gina, "Avoiding Mammogram Guidelines," *New York Times,* Dec. 5, 1993.
84. Kolata, Gina, "Mammograms Before 50? A Hung Jury," *New York Times,* Nov. 24, 1993.
85. Kolata, Gina, "Value of Mammograms Before 50 Debated Anew," *New York Times,* Dec. 16, 1992.
86. Ibid.
87. Ibid.
88. Ibid.
89. "Ten Facts About Breast Cancer That May Surprise You," The Breast Cancer Fund, San Francisco, CA.
90. Ibid.
91. "Mammography: Investigation," *ABC News—Prime-time Live,* Feb. 27, 1991.
92. "Medical Malpractice Law," *Good Morning America,* Aug. 29, 1991.
93. "Woman Wins $2.7 Million for Mistaken Mastectomy," Associated Press (*Sarasota Herald-Tribune),* April 20, 1994.

94. "Mammography: Investigation," *ABC News—Prime-time Live,* Feb. 27, 1991.

95. McDougall, John, M.D., *McDougall's Medicine: A Challenging Second Opinion,* New Century, Piscat-away, NJ, 1985.

96. "Mammogram Interpretations Are Questioned in a Report," *New York Times,* Dec. 2, 1994

97. Taylor, Paul, "Mammogram Study Sparks Controversy," *Globe and Mail,* Nov. 14, 1992.

98. McDougall, John, M.D., *McDougall's Medicine: A Challenging Second Opinion,* New Century, Piscataway, NJ, 1985.

99. McDougall, John, M.D., and McDougall, Mary, *The McDougall Plan,* New Century, Piscataway, NJ, 1983.

100. Kolata, Gina, "New Ability to Find Earliest Cancers: A Mixed Blessing?" *New York Times,* Nov. 8, 1994.

101. "Today in America," MSNBC, July 6, 1999.

102. *Oprah Winfrey Show,* Aug. 1, 1994.

103. Dowling, Claudia G., "Fighting Back," *LIFE,* May 1994.

104. Kolata, Gina, "Weighing Spending on Breast Cancer Research," *New York Times,* Oct. 20, 1993.

105. Starlanyl, Devin J., M.D., and Copeland, Mary Ellen, M.S., M.A., *Fibromyalgia & Chronic Myofascial Pain Syndrome,* New Harbinger Publications, CA, 1996.

106. Andrews, Marcia, and Robert B. Cooper, eds., *Everything You Need to Know About Diseases,* Spring-house Publishing, 1997.

107. Anthony, Catherine P., *Textbook of Anatomy and Physiology,* Mosby, St. Louis, 1959.

108. Stolberg, Sheryl Gay, "Officials: Risk from Medicines Growing," *New York Times*, June 3, 1999.

109. Ibid.

110. Ibid.

111. Ibid.

112. Ibid.

113. Yanick, P., *Townsend Letter for Doctors,* pp. 88–91, Jan. 1999.

114. The Surgeon General's "Report on Nutrition and Health," U.S. Department of Health and Human Services, 1988.

115. Welch, C., "Cinocoronary Arteriography in Young Men," *Circulation,* No. 42, 1970; p. I., "Prediction of Coronary Heart Disease Based on Clinical Suspicion, Age, Total Cholesterol and Triglycerides," *Circulation,* No. 42, 1970; Zampogna, A., "Relationship Between Lipids and Occlusive Coronary Artery Disease," *Annals of Internal Medicine,* No. 84, 1976; Jenkins, P., "Severity of Coronary Atherosclerosis Related to Lipoprotein Concentration," *British Medical Journal,* No. 2, 1978; Pocock, S., "Concentrations of High-Density Lipoprotein Cholesterol, Triglycerides

and Total Cholesterol in Ischemic Heart Disease," *British Medical Journal*, No. 298, 1989; Rosengren, A., "Impact of Cardiovascular Risk Factors on Coronary Heart Disease and Mortality Among Middle-Aged Diabetic Men, A General Population Study," *British Medical Journal*, No. 299, 1989; Pekkanen, J., "Risk Factors and 25-Year Risk of Coronary Heart Disease: The Finnish Cohorts of the Seven Country Study," *British Medical Journal*, No. 299, 1989; Benfante, R., "Is Elevated Serum Cholesterol Level a Risk Factor for Coronary Heart Disease in the Elderly? *Journal of the American Medical Association*, No. 269, 1990; Castelli, W., "Epidemiology of Coronary Heart Disease: The Framingham Study," *American Journal of Medicine*, No. 76, 1984; Kannel, W., "Cholesterol in the Prediction of Atherosclerotic Disease: New Perspectives Based on the Framingham Study," *Annals of Internal Medicine*, No. 90, 1979; Stamler, J., "Is the Relationship Between Serum Cholesterol and Risk of Premature Death from Coronary Heart Disease Continuous and Graded?" *Journal of the American Medical Association*, No. 256, 1986; Connor, W., "The Key Role of Nutritional Factors in the Prevention of Coronary Heart Disease," *Preventive Medicine*, No. 1, 1972; Pritikin, N., *The Pritikin Program for Diet and Exercise*, Grosset & Dunlap, New York, 1979; McDougall, J., *McDougall's Medicine: A Challenging Second Opinion*, New Century, Piscataway, NJ, 1985; Ornish, D., *Dr. Dean Ornish's Program for Reversing Heart Disease*, Random House, New York, 1990; Whitaker, J., *Reversing Heart Disease*, Warner, New York, 1985; Connor, W., "Serum Lipids in Men Receiving High Cholesterol and Cholesterol-Free Diets," *Journal of Clinical Investigation*, No. 40, 1961; Imai, H., "Angiotoxicity of Oxygenated Sterols and Possible Precursors," *Science*, No. 207, 1980; Keys, A., "Lessons from Serum Cholesterol Studies in Japan, Hawaii and Los Angeles," *Annals of Internal Medicine*, No. 48, 1958; Levy, R.I., "Declining Mortality in Coronary Heart Disease," *Arteriosclerosis*, No. 1, Sept./Oct. 1981; Shekelle, R.B., "Diet, Serum Cholesterol and Death from Coronary Heart Disease," *New England Journal of Medicine*, No. 304, 1981; Wissler, R.W., "Studies of Progression of Advanced Atherosclerosis in Experimental Animals and Man," *Annals of New York Academy of Science*, No. 275, 1976; Samuel, P., "Further Validation of the Plasma Isotope Ratio Method for Measurement of Cholesterol Absorption In Man," *Journal of Lipid Research*, No. 23, 1982; Insull, W., "Cholesterol, Triglyceride and Phospho-lipid Content of Intima, Media and Atherosclerotic Fatty Streaks in Human Thoracic Aorta," *Journal of Clinical Investigation*, No. 45, 1966; Katz, S., "Physical Chemistry of the Lipids of Human Atherosclerotic Lesions: Demonstration of a Lesion Intermediate Between Fatty Streaks and Advanced Plaques," *Journal of Clinical Investigation*, No. 58, 1976; Proudfit, W., "Selective Cine Coronary Arteriography: Correlation with Clinical Findings in 1,000 Patients," *Circulation*, No. |

33, 1966; Blankenhorn, D.H., et al., "Dietary Fat Influences Human Coronary Lesion Formation," *Circulation,* No. 78 (Supp. II), 1988; Brown, E.G., et al., "Arteriographic Assessment of Coronary Arteriosclerosis, Review of Current Methods, Their Limitations, and Clinical Applications," *Arteriosclerosis,* No. 2, 1982; Gould, K.L., et al., "Improvement of Stenosis Geometry by Quantitative Coronary Arteriography After Adequate Cholesterol Lowering in Man," *Circulation,* No. 80, 1989; Leaf, A., "Management of Hypercholesterolemia," *New England Journal of Medicine,* No. 321, 1989; Shekelle, R.B., "Dietary Cholesterol and Ischemic Heart Disease," *Lancet,* No. 1 (8648), 1989.

116. Sorenson, Marc, *Mega-Health,* Sorenson, Ivins, Utah, 1993.

117. "Heart Disease Facts." Centers for Disease Control and Prevention, *Centers for Disease Control and Prevention*, 2 Dec. 2019, www.cdc.gov/heartdisease/ facts.htm.

118. Glick, D., "New Age Meets Hippocrates," *Newsweek,* July 13, 1992.

119. "Second Opinions for Bypass Surgery," *Health & Healing,* Vol. 2, No. 1, Jan. 1992.

120. Sorenson, Marc, *Mega-Health,* Sorenson, Ivins, Utah, 1993.

121. "Smokers Have a Higher Breast Cancer Death Risk," *New York Times,* May 25, 1994.

122. McMurray, M., "The Absorption of Cholesterol and the Sterol Balance in the Tarahumara Indians of Mexico Fed Cholesterol-free and High Cholesterol Diets," *American Journal of Clinical Nutrition,* No. 41, 1985; Wells, V., "Egg Yolk and Serum Cholesterol Levels: The Importance of Dietary Cholesterol In-take," *British Medical Journal,* No. 1, 1963.

123. Connor, W., "The Interrelated Effects of Dietary Cholesterol and Fat Upon Human Serum Lipid Levels," *Journal of Clinical Investigation,* No. 43, 1964.

124. McDougall, John, M.D., *McDougall's Medicine: A Challenging Second Opinion,* New Century, Piscataway, NJ, 1985.

125. Ibid.

126. Willit, W.C., et al., "Relation of Meat, Fat and Fiber Intake to the Risk of Colon Cancer in a Prospective Study Among Women," *New England Journal of Medicine,* No. 323, 1990; Whittemore, A.S., et al., "Diet, Physical Activity and Colorectal Cancer Among Chinese in North America and China," *Journal of the National Cancer Institute,* No. 82, 1990.

127. Kolata, G., "Animal Fat Is Tied to Colon Cancer," *New York Times,* Dec. 13, 1990.

128. Katsuoyanni, K., "Diet and Breast Cancer: A Case-Control Study in Greece," *International Journal of Cancer,* No. 38, 1986.

129. "Council Urges Major Changes for U.S. Diets," *Los Angeles Times,* March 2, 1989.

130. Lea, A., "Dietary Factors Associated with Death Rates from Certain Neoplasms in Man," *Lancet,* No. 2, 1966; Caroll, K., "Experimental Evidence

of Dietary Factors and Hormone-Dependent Cancers, *Cancer Research,* No. 35, 1975; Drasar, B., "Environ-mental Factors and Cancer of the Colon and Breast," *British Journal of Cancer,* No. 27, 1973; Armstrong, B., "Environmental Factors and Cancer Incidence and Mortality in Different Countries With Special Reference to Dietary Practices," *International Journal of Cancer,* No. 15, 1975; Knox, E., "Foods and Diseases," *British Journal of Cancer,* No. 31, 1977; Hiryama, T., "Epidemiology of Breast Cancer with Special Reference to the Role of Diet," *Preventive Medicine,* No. 7, 1978; Gray, G., "Breast Cancer Incidence and Mortality Rates in Relation to Known Factors and Dietary Practices," *British Journal of Cancer,* No. 39, 1979; Hems, G., "The Contributions of Diet and Childbearing to Breast Cancer," *British Journal of Cancer,* No. 37, 1978; Howe, G., "A Cohort Study of Fat Intake and Risk of Breast Cancer," *Journal of the National Cancer Institute,* No. 83, 1991; Henderson, M., "Cancer Incidence in Seattle Wom-en's Health Trial Participants by Group and Time Since Randomization," *Journal of the National Cancer Institute,* No. 83, 1991; Yu, S., "A Case-Controlled Study of Dietary and Non-Dietary Risk Factors for Breast Cancer in Shanghai," *Cancer Research,* No. 50, 1990; Van't Veer, P., "Dietary Fat and the Risk of Breast Cancer," *International Journal of Epidemiology,* No. 19, 1990; Willett, W., "The Search for the Causes of Breast and Colon Cancer," *Nature,* No. 338, 1989; Berrino, F., "Mediterranean Diet and Cancer," *Euro-pean Journal of Clinical Nutrition,* No. 43 (Supp. 2), 1989; Howe, G., "Dietary Factors and Risk of Breast Cancer: Combined Analysis of 12 Case-Controlled Studies," *Journal of the National Cancer Institute,* No. 82, 1990; Brisson, J., "Diet, Mammographic Features of Breast Tissue, and Breast Cancer Risk," *American Journal of Epidemiology,* No. 130, 1989; Foniolo, P., "Calorie-Providing Nutrients and Risk of Breast Cancer," *Journal of the National Cancer Institute,* No. 81, 1989.

131. Raloff, Janet, "EcoCancers," *Science News*, Vol. 144, No. 1, July 3, 1993.

132. Goldin, B., "The Relationship Between Estrogen Levels and Diets of Caucasian-American and Oriental-Immigrant Women," *American Journal of Clinical Nu-trition*, No. 44, 1986.

133. Schultz, T., "Nutrient Intake and Hormonal Status of Premenopausal Vegetarian," *Nutrition and Cancer,* No. 4, 1983.

134. Bennet, F., "Diet and Sex-Hormone Concentrations: An Intervention Study for the Type of Fat Consumed," *American Journal of Clinical Nutrition,* No. 52, 1990; Woods, M., "Low-Fat, High-Fiber Diet and Serum Estrone Sulfate in Premenopausal Women," *American Journal of Clinical Nutrition,* No. 49, 1989; Rose, D., "Effect of a Low-Fat Diet on Hormone Levels in Women with Cystic Breast Disease," *Journal of the National Cancer Institute,* No. 78, 1987; Rose, D., "Effect of a Low-Fat

Diet on Hormone Levels in Women with Cystic Breast Disease, II. Serum Radio-immunoassayable Prolactin and Growth Hormone and Bioactive Lactogenic Hormones," *Journal of the National Cancer Institute,* No. 78, 1987; Gorbach, S., "Estrogens, Breast Cancer and Intestinal Flora," *Review of Infectious Diseases,* No. 6 (Supp. 1), 1984.

135. Ellerbee, Linda, "The Other Epidemic—What Every Woman Needs to Know About Breast Cancer," ABC-TV, Sept. 14, 1993; Frommer, D., "Changing Age of Menopause," *British Medical Journal,* No. 2, 1964; Trichopolulos, D., "Menopause and Breast Cancer Risk," *Journal of the National Cancer Institute,* No. 48, 1972; Armstrong, B., "Diet and Reproductive Hor-mones, A Study of Vegetarian and Non-Vegetarian Postmenopausal Women," *Journal of the National Cancer Institute,* No. 67, 1981; Hill, P., "Environmental Factors of Breast and Prostatic Cancer," *Cancer Research,* No. 41, 1981.

136. "Breast Cancer—Complacency Is the Enemy of Cure," *FDA Consumer,* July/Aug. 1991.

137. Kagawa, Y., "Impact of Westernization on the Nutrition of the Japanese: Changes in Physique, Cancer, Longevity and Centenarians," *Preventive Medicine,* No. 7, 1978; Haenzel, W., "Studies of Japanese Migrants, I. Mortality from Cancer and Other Diseases Among Japanese in the U.S.," *Journal of the National Cancer Institute,* No. 40, 1968; Kolonel, L., "Nutrient Intakes in Relation to Cancer Incidence in Hawaii," *British Journal of Cancer,* No. 44, 1981; Buell, P., "Changing Incidence of Breast Cancer in Japanese-American Women," *Journal of the National Cancer Institute,* No. 51, 1973; Wynder, E., "Strategies Toward the Primary Prevention of Cancer," *Archives of Surgery,* No. 125, 1990.

138. Powell, Bill, and Myers, Patrick S., "Death by Fried Chicken," *Newsweek,* Sept. 24, 1990.

139. "Fat Poses Dual Threat of Breast Cancer," *Science News,* Vol. 138, No. 19, Nov. 10, 1990.

140. Angier, Natalie, "Chemists Learn Why Vegetables Are Good for You," *New York Times,* April 13, 1993.

141. Yeager, Selene, "FOOD: The Ultimate Protector," *New York Times,* Jan. 18, 1999.

142. Recer, Paul, "Broccoli Extract Shown to Block Breast Cancer," The Associated Press (*Sarasota Herald-Tribune),* April 12, 1994.

143. Lem, Sharon, "OJ Fights Breast Cancer," *Toronto Sun,* Aug. 7, 1997.

144. Carper, Jean, *Food—Your Miracle Medicine,* HarperCollins, New York, 1993.

145. Ibid.

146. Kritchevsky, David, Ph.D., "Nutrition and Breast Cancer," *Cancer,* Vol. 66, No. 6, Sept. 15, 1990.

147. Howe, Geoffrey R., Ph.D., et al., "Dietary Factors and the Risk of Breast Cancer: Combined Analysis of 12 Case-Controlled Studies," *Journal of the National Cancer Institute,* No. 82, 1990.

148. McKeown, L.A., "Diet High in Fruits and Vegetables Linked to Lower Breast Cancer Risk," *Medical Tribune,* July 9, 1992.

149. "Strong Views on Origins of Cancer," *New York Times,* July 5, 1994.

150. Ibid.

151. Ibid.

152. "Low-Fat Diet Slows a Cancer in Mice, Study Says," *New York Times,* October 4, 1995.

153. Power, Lawrence, M.D., "Lowering the Risk of Breast Cancer," *Los Angeles Times,* Dec. 4, 1984.

154. "Personal Health," *New York Times,* Feb. 16, 1994.

155. *New England Journal of Medicine,* Oct. 24, 1985.

156. "Fighting Cancer—Are We Doing Enough?" CNN Newsmaker, Sunday, July 7, 1991.

157. Holland, Jimmie, M.D., "Cancer Do's—Cancer Don'ts," *Health Confidential,* Vol. 7, No. 12, Dec. 1993.

158. "New Risks for Meat Eaters," *Science News,* Vol. 146, No. 3, July 16, 1994.

159. "Conflicting Advice in Breast Cancer," *Nightline,* March 19, 1993.

160. Chalmers, Irena, *The Great Food Almanac—A Feast of Facts from A to Z,* HarperCollins, San Francisco, 1994.

161. Campbell, T. Colin, M.D., et al., "Cornell-Oxford-China Project on Nutrition, Health and Environment, Diet, Lifestyle and Mortality in China: A Study of the Characteristics of 65 Countries," Oxford University Press, The China People's Medical Publishing House, 1990.

162. "Huge Study of Diet Indicts Fat and Meats," *New York Times,* May 8, 1990.

163. Mead, Nathaniel, "The Champion Diet," *East-West Journal,* Vol. 20, No. 9, Sept. 1990.

164. Regan, Tom, "But for the Sake of Some Little Mouthful of Flesh," *The Animals Agenda,* No. 1, Feb. 1989; U.S. Dept. of Agriculture, Agriculture Statistics, 1988.

165. *Eat for Life: The Food & Nutrition Board's Guide to Re-ducing Your Risk of Chronic Disease,* National Academy Press, Washington, D.C., 1992.

166. Hellmich, Nanci, "In Healthful Living, East Beats West," *USA Today,* June 6, 1990.

167. Sherman, H., "Calcium Requirements of Maintenance in Man," *Journal of Biological Chemistry,* No. 44, 1920.

168. Bresala, N., "Relationships of Animal Protein-Rich Diet to Kidney Stone Formation and Calcium Metabolism," *Journal of Clinical Endocri-*

nology and Metabolism, No. 66, 1988; Zemel, M., "Calcium Utilization: Effect of Varying Level and Source of Dietary Protein," *American Journal of Clinical Nutrition,* No. 48, 1988.

169. Lewinnek, G.E., "The Significance and a Compara-tive Analysis of the Epidemiology of Hip Fractures," *Clinical Orthopedics and Related Research,* Vol. 152, Oct. 1980; Solomon, L., "Osteoporosis and Fracture of the Femoral Neck in the South African Bantu," *Journal of Bone and Joint Surgery,* Vol. 50B, Feb. 1968; United Nations Food and Agriculture Organization, *FAO Production Yearbook,* Vol. 37, 1984, and *Food Balance Sheets,* 1979–1981 Average; Walter, A., "The Human Requirement of Calcium: Should Low Intakes Be Supplemented?," *American Journal of Clinical Nutrition,* Vol. 25, May 1972; Walker, A., "Osteoporosis and Calcium Deficiency," *American Journal of Clinical Nutrition,* Vol. 16, March 1965.

170. "Consensus Conference: Osteoporosis," *Journal of the American Medical Association,* No. 252, 1984.

171. Campbell, T. Colin, M.D., et al., "Cornell-Oxford-China Project on Nutrition, Health and Environment, Diet, Lifestyle and Mortality in China: A Study of the Characteristics of 65 Countries," Oxford University Press, The China People's Medical Publishing House, 1990; "Huge Study of Diet Indicts Fat and Meats," *New York Times,* May 8, 1990.

172. Ibid.

173. Abdulla, M., "Nutrient Intake and Health Status of Vegans, Chemical Analysis of Diets Using the Duplicate Portion Sampling Technique," *American Journal of Clinical Nutrition,* No. 34, 1981; Ellis, F., "Veganism, Clinical Findings and Investigations," *American Journal of Clinical Nutrition,* No. 23, 1970; Sanders, T., "Hematological Studies on Vegans," *British Medical Journal,* No. 40, 1978; Anderson, B., "The Iron and Zinc Status of Long-Term Vegetarian Women," *American Journal of Clinical Nutrition,* No. 34, 1981.

174. Sorenson, Marc, *Mega-Health,* Sorenson, Ivins, Utah, 1993.

175. Campbell, T. Colin, M.D., et al., "Cornell-Oxford-China Project on Nutrition, Health and Environment, Diet, Lifestyle and Mortality in China: A Study of the Characteristics of 65 Countries," Oxford University Press, The China People's Medical Publishing House, 1990; "Huge Study of Diet Indicts Fat and Meats," *New York Times,* May 8, 1990.

176. Ibid.

177. Dowling, Claudia G., "Fighting Back," *LIFE,* May 1994.

178. Campbell, T. Colin, M.D., et al., "Cornell-Oxford-China Project on Nutrition, Health and Environment, Diet, Lifestyle and Mortality in China: A Study of the Characteristics of 65 Countries," Oxford University Press, The China People's Medical Publishing House, 1990; "Huge Study of Diet Indicts Fat and Meats," *New York Times,* May 8, 1990.

179. Chalmers, Irena, *The Great Food Almanac—A Feast of Facts from A to Z,* HarperCollins, San Francisco, 1994.
180. Hellmich, Nanci, "In Healthful Living, East Beats West," *USA Today,* June 6, 1990.
181. Ibid.
182. Mead, Nathaniel, "The Champion Diet," *East-West Journal,* Vol. 20, No. 9, Sept. 1990.
183. "Position Paper of the American Dietetic Association: Vegetarian Diets—Technical Support Paper," *Journal of the American Dietetic Association,* Vol. Ii, No. 3, March 1988.
184. As cited in *Vegetarian Times,* Feb. 1991.
185. Seely, Rod R., Ph.D., Stephens, Trent D., Ph.D., Tate, Phillip, D.A., *Anatomy & Physiology,* Mosby, St. Louis, 1992.
186. Blair, S.N., et al., "Physical Fitness and All Cause Mortality: A Prospective Study of Health: Men and Women," *Journal of the American Medical Association,* Vol. 262, No. 17, Nov. 3, 1989.
187. Seely, Rod R., Ph.D., Stephens, Trent D., Ph.D., Tate, Phillip, D.A., *Anatomy & Physiology,* Mosby, St. Louis, 1992.
188. Blair, S.N., et al., "Physical Fitness and All Cause Mortality: A Prospective Study of Health: Men and Women," *Journal of the American Medical Association,* Vol. 262, No. 17, Nov. 3, 1989.
189. Koplan, J.P., et al., "Physical Activity, Physical Fitness, and Health: Time to Act," *Journal of the American Medical Association,* Vol. 262, No. 17, Nov. 3, 1991; Conversation with Dan Kaser of National Sporting Goods Association, Nov. 12, 1991.
190. Rippe, J.M., *Dr. James M. Rippe's Complete Book of Fitness Walking,* Prentice-Hall, New York, 1989.
191. Ibid.
192. Ibid.
193. Ibid.
194. "Progress Toward Achieving the 1990 National Objectives for Physical Fitness and Exercise," Centers for Disease Control, MMWR No. 38, 1989.
195. "Leisure-Time Physical Activity Levels and Risk of Coronary Heart Disease and Death," *Journal of the American Medical Association,* No. 258, 1987.
196. Wiley, C., "Walk This Way," *Vegetarian Times,* Jan. 1992.
197. Ibid.
198. Koplan, J.P., et al., "Physical Activity, Physical Fitness, and Health: Time to Act," *Journal of the American Medical Association,* Vol. 262, No. 17, Nov. 3, 1991.
199. Gavin, J., *The Exercise Habit,* Human Kinetics Publishing, 1992, as quoted in *Bottom Line,* Vol. 13, No. 14, July 30, 1992.
200. "Study Links Exercise to Drop in Breast Cancer," *New York Times,* Sept. 21, 1994.

201. Bazell, Robert, *NBC Network News,* Sept. 20, 1994.
202. Kolata, Gina, "Study Bolsters Idea That Exercise Cuts Breast Cancer Risk," *New York Times,* May 1, 1997.
203. "A.M. Exercisers Stay with It," *Aviation Medical Bulletin,* Dec. 1990.
204. Rippe, J.M., *Dr. James M. Rippe's Complete Book of Fitness Walking,* Prentice-Hall, New York, 1989.
205. Ibid.
206. Ibid.
207. Ibid.
208. Ibid.
209. Ibid.
210. Hottinger, B., "Walking Your Way to Fitness," *Vegetarian Voice,* Vol. 18, No. 4.
211. Study Conducted at the Veterans' Affairs Medical Center, Salt Lake City, reported in *Bottom Line,* Vol. 12, No. 19, Oct. 15, 1991.
212. Study by David Nieman, Exercise Physiologist, reported in *Bottom Line,* Vol. 12, No. 21, Nov. 15, 1991.
213. *The Wellness Encyclopedia,* University of California, Berkeley Wellness Letter, Houghton Mifflin, Boston, 1991.
214. Wiley, C., "Walk This Way," *Vegetarian Times,* Jan. 1992.
215. Study headed by James R. White, Ph.D., Director of the Exercise Physiology and Human Performance Lab at the University of California, San Diego, reported in *Bottom Line,* Vol. 12, No. 12, June 30, 1991.
216. Data from Betty Kamen, Ph.D., writing in "Let's Live," reported in *Bottom Line,* Vol. 13, No. 1, Jan. 15, 1992.
217. Rippe, J.M., *Dr. James M. Rippe's Complete Book of Fitness Walking,* Prentice-Hall, New York, 1989; Wiley, C., "Walk This Way," *Vegetarian Times,* Jan. 1992; Hottinger, B., "Walking Your Way to Fitness," *Vegetarian Voice,* Vol. 18, No. 4.
218. Wiley, C., "Walk This Way," *Vegetarian Times,* Jan. 1992.
219. Ibid.
220. Carter, Albert E., "The Miracles of Rebound Exer-cises," National Institute of Reboundology & Health, Edmonds, WA, 1979.
221. Leahy, M., "Can This Man Help You Live to 140?" *Los Angeles Magazine,* April 1983.
222. Trichopoulou, Antonia, "Consumption of Olive Oil and Specific Food Groups in Relation to Breast Cancer Risk in Greece," *Journal of the National Cancer Institute,* Vol. 87, No. 2, Jan. 18, 1995.
223. Osborn, T., "Amino Acids in Nutrition and Growth," *Journal of Biological Chemistry,* No. 17, 1914.
224. Clinton, S., "The Vegetarian Perspective—An Examination of Nutrition Education and the American Diet," *Vegetarian Journal,* Vol. 9, No. 3, May/June 1990.
225. Ibid.

226. Ibid.
227. Ibid.
228. "U.S.D.A. Cancels Nutrition Chart: Who's Being Served?" *New York Times,* May 8, 1991; U.S.D.A. Wilts Under Pressure, Kills New Food Group Pyramid," *Washington Post,* April 27, 1991.
229. Ibid.
230. "U.S.D.A. Cancels Nutrition Chart: Who's Being Served?" *New York Times,* May 8, 1991; U.S.D.A. Wilts Under Pressure, Kills New Food Group Pyramid," *Washington Post,* April 27, 1991.
231. Nesmith, J., "Pyramid's Something to Chew On," Cox News Service (*Sarasota Herald-Tribune*), April 29, 1992.
232. Trichopoulou, Antonia, "Consumption of Olive Oil and Specific Food Groups in Relation to Breast Cancer Risk in Greece," *Journal of the National Cancer Institute,* Vol. 87, No. 2, Jan. 18, 1995.
233. "Fear of Fat," CBS-TV, *48 Hours,* Oct. 9, 1994.
234. Cousins, N., *Anatomy of an Illness,* Norton, New York, 1979.
235. Talan, J., "Good Thoughts—Good Health," *Sarasota Herald-Tribune,* June 12, 1991.
236. Chopra, D., *Quantum Healing,* Bantam, New York, 1989.
237. Frank, J.O., *Persuasion and Healing: A Comparative Study of Psychotherapy,* Johns Hopkins University Press, Baltimore, 1973.
238. Chopra, D., *Quantum Healing,* Bantam, New York, 1989.
239. Cushing, H., *The Life of Sir William Osler,* Oxford University Press, New York, 1940.
240. Shelton, Herbert M., *Natural Hygiene: Man's Pristine Way of Life,* Dr. Shelton's Health School, TX, 1968.
241. Benson, H., "The Placebo Effect," *Journal of the American Medical Association,* Vol. 232, No. 12, June 23, 1975; Booth, G., "Psychobiological Aspects of Spontaneous Regressions of Cancer," *Journal of the American Academy of Psychoanalysis,* Vol. 1, No. 3, 1973; Everson, T.C., et al., *Spontaneous Regression of Cancer,* Philadelphia, 1966; Simonton, O.C., *Getting Well Again,* Tarcher, New York, 1978; Anderson, R.A., *Dr. Robert A. Anderson's Comprehensive Guide to Wellness Medicine,* Keats, CT, 1987.
242. Vaux, K., "Religion and Health, *Preventive Medicine,* Vol. 5, No. 4, Dec. 1976; Seventh-Day Adventist Mortality Study, 1958-1965, School of Health, Loma Linda University, CA.
243. Oberleder, M., *Avoid the Aging Trap,* Acropolis, Wash-ington, D.C., 1982.
244. Beecher, H.D., "Surgery as Placebo," *Journal of the American Medical Association,* Vol. 176, No. 13, July 1, 1961.
245. Klopfer, B., "Psychological Variables in Human Cancer," *Journal of Projective Techniques,* Vol. 21, No. 4, Dec. 1957.
246. Beecher, H.K., "The Powerful Placebo," *Journal of the American Medical Association,* Vol. 159, No. 17, Dec. 29, 1955; Wolf, S., "The Pharma-

cology of Placebos," *Pharmacology Review,* Vol. 11, No. 4, Dec. 1959; Pogge, R., "The Toxic Placebo: Side and Toxic Effects Reported During Administration of Placebo Medicine," *Medical Times,* No. 91, Aug. 1963.

247. Brown, S., "Side Reactions to Pyribenzamine Medication," *Proclamation of the Society of Experimental Biological Medicine,* Vol. 67, No. 3, March 1948.

248. Goleman, Daniel, "Placebo Effect Is Shown to Be Twice as Powerful as Expected," *New York Times,* Aug. 17, 1993.

249. Ibid.

250. Chopra, D., *Unconditional Life,* Bantam, New York, 1991.

251. Wright, K., "Going by the Numbers," *New York Times Magazine,* Dec. 15, 1991.

252. Ibid.

253. Ibid.

254. Becnel, T., "Looking to the Future," *Sarasota Herald-Tribune,* Dec. 18, 1991.

APPENDIX I

The Magic of Water

The most enduring image of humanity's exploration of space has turned out to be the sight of a small blue pearl of a planet orbiting a rather ordinary star in an out-of-the-way corner of the galaxy. From space, the blue color of our planet distinguishes it from anything else as far as our telescopes can see. The Hubble Space Telescope can take pictures trillions of miles in any direction, but our little blue pearl is the only one in sight.

What makes our planet so unique, special, and extraordinary? Water not only colors our world but also provides it with the capacity to harbor life. Water is Nature's catalyst, the key to life. There are places on Earth that are so dry, parched, and inhospitable looking that you would think no life could possibly be sustained there. Then along comes a life-giving rain and a dazzling spectacle of transformation occurs. In a few short days there is a lush carpet of plants and flowers, a circus of colors as far as the eye can see where there was nothing but parched and cracked earth. Animals by the thousands seem to appear out of nowhere to feast on the bounty.

WATER IS NOT "JUST" WATER

Recognizing the uniqueness of our planet and the primary role water plays in our life and our health rightly makes us view water in a new, more reverential way. We honor the miracle of life when we acknowledge the incalculable importance of water and strive to grasp the full measure of the fundamental role it plays in our health and fitness.

Just as water is the key to life and the health of our planet, it is a primary key to our personal health and well-being. In seeking vibrant health for ourselves and our loved ones, we would be well advised to educate ourselves about water. With advanced technology and water science, water is not "just" water anymore: a new generation of hydration and modified, enhanced, and restructured waters have been designed to take us beyond surviving to thriving as healthy, high-performance individuals. These innovations will have a profound effect on our national and global health in the years to come.

WATER BEINGS OF THE WATER PLANET

In looking at our blue planet it quickly becomes apparent that most of its surface, in fact, about 70 percent, is water. I don't know why it is called planet Earth; clearly it should be called planet Water. A most interesting fact to ponder is that our bodies are also approximately 70 percent water. We are, in the most literal sense possible, water beings living on a water planet. Our body fluids are an internal ocean that regulates and drives all bodily functions much the way water and water cycles govern organic life on the Earth.

As we make our way through the journey of life, there is no

gift that is more desired or more cherished than good health. Some might say that wealth is desired more, but what good is money if you're too sick to enjoy what it can buy? It is impossible to discuss the great gift of health without considering the role of water in acquiring and maintaining it—no more than one could discuss the nature of a majestic 200-foot redwood tree without mentioning the soil in which it grows.

NEW THINKING ABOUT HEALTH AND WATER

In striving for the highest attainable level of health, we are helped by an awareness that the two most extensive systems in the living body, the cardiovascular and lymph systems, work hand in hand in an untiring effort to keep the body healthy. The cardiovascular system has the heart at its center. The heart pumps six quarts of blood through an amazing 90,000 miles of blood vessels that bring oxygen to every cell of the body. Keeping this system in top condition is extremely important because cardiovascular disease takes more lives than all other causes of death by disease combined.

The lymph system, as has been discussed, is the backbone of the immune system. As you have learned, the body is constantly generating wastes, or toxins, both from the billions of spent cells that die every day and from the residue of the 70 tons of food we each eat in our lifetimes. If these toxins were produced in our body unchecked, we would quickly be ushered to the grave; they are the underlying cause of arthritis, fibromyalgia, lupus, and chronic fatigue syndrome. It is the job of the lymph system—which contains three times more lymph fluid than the body does blood—to gather up these toxins from every cell in the body, break them down, and remove them.

It is the activities of the cardiovascular and the lymph systems that determines how long we will live and how healthy we will be. No matter what your health goals are—to lose weight, increase energy, remove pain, overcome or prevent disease—you can be absolutely certain that nothing will be achieved without the constant and tireless efforts of these two systems.

"What," you may be asking, "do the cardiovascular system and lymph system have to do with the discussion of water?" Just this: blood, the medium of the cardiovascular system, and lymph fluid, the medium of the lymph system, are both 90 percent water, but water with a distinct composition. We call it *plasma*. But the need for water doesn't stop with the cardiovascular and lymph systems. There are trillions of other activities performed by the living body every moment. Consider the amniotic fluid that envelopes and protects a fetus. Saliva is almost all water; without it your tongue would stick to the inside of your mouth—you wouldn't be able to swallow. The fluid that moistens the eye so that it can move with ease, as well as tears, are both mostly water. If not for water, food would not be digested as digestive juices are practically all water. In fact, without the fluid that surrounds all the internal organs of the body the organs would stick together and tear. And of course, the connective tissue is also mostly water. All the joints of the body move with such ease because of synovial fluid which is 90 percent water; without it the joints quickly become susceptible to arthritis. Even our bones are 35 percent water. We are water beings!

> *"Water is . . . not necessary to life, but rather life itself."*
> —Antoine de Saint-Exupéry

Remove all water from the human body and what is left would fit into a shoebox. When you consider that water is second only to air as a requirement of staying alive, it's shocking how few people recognize the devastating repercussions to the body when it is insufficiently hydrated and, conversely, the immeasurable good that comes from properly meeting all the body's water needs.

It's also surprising that many people fail to realize how much water is lost from the body every day. As a water being on a water planet the human body is constructed so that there is an unceasing, round-the-clock ebb and flow of water in and out of it. Every day each of us loses about two quarts of water through both perspiration and respiration. Depending upon variables, such as physical activity and diet, we can easily lose twice that amount or more.

The skin contains millions of pores, which constantly secrete moisture. Obviously, when exercise or physical activity is heightened we perspire more heavily and can see the loss of water, but there is not a moment, day or night, that our skin is not excreting some water. We also lose water every time we exhale. Breathe on a mirror or window and you can see the moisture from your lungs on the glass. Since you exhale many thousands of times a day, and each time you do you lose some water, you can lose a third of a quart or more per day.

This water must be replaced every day and failing to do so will cause you harm. Depriving the body of its water needs, intentionally or unintentionally, can have catastrophic results that affect its every activity and function. No matter what your health goals are, all are sabotaged by shortchanging the body of its water needs. And as you will learn, the water-modifying and -enhancing minerals, trace elements, and complex organic molecules play a profound role in their synergy with water.

GET HYDRATED! GET HEALTHY!

I have been studying and teaching the principles of a healthy lifestyle for 35 of my 60 years on Earth. I have seen many ironies relating to people's quest to live a pain-free life of health and well-being. I can tell you from experience that perhaps the most tragic irony of all is the one associated with the pain, ill-health, and disease that afflict so many people who could have avoided it all if only they had done something as simple and natural as properly hydrating their body. "Normal" aging is often described as a continuous process characterized by a decrease in lean body mass, an increase in fat, and a decrease in hydration—but I want to show my readers how to side-step such "normality."

It has been said that one of the greatest threats to the survival of any animal, including man, is that of dehydration. Yet millions of people continue to scramble around trying all manner of remedies in order to recapture or maintain their health. They resort to drugs that are inherently toxic and dangerous, and all too frequently result in death. They take fistfuls of supplements, most of them synthesized in a laboratory or extracted with chemicals or heat, both of which compromise their worth. They go on diets that are only temporary at best and, in the case of fad diets, stress the body. And of course there is no shortage of expensive treatments all designed to force the body into doing what it would have done for itself automatically if only it wasn't sabotaged by insufficient hydration.

For whatever reason, people have failed to recognize the immeasurable benefit they could reap simply by replenishing the water they lose every day and properly hydrating their body. This alone would significantly optimize the body's own healing capabilities, which would in turn dramatically improve a person's health and well-being.

I say this is tragic because even though there is something so natural and uncomplicated as simply providing the living body with the water it must have to survive and thus improve health, there are estimates that as many as 75 percent of the population are underhydrated, many of them chronically. There are actually significant numbers of people who drink no water at all. As embarrassed as I am to say it, there was a time in my early life when I was one of them. My attitude was, why drink water when I could have a Dr Pepper instead? And believe me when I tell you that my health suffered as a result, even though I didn't know it at the time.

People have told me that instead of water they drink coffee, soda, or pasteurized bottled juices. What they don't realize is that every one of these results in acidity in the body and is counterproductive because it doesn't properly hydrate the cells. They drink these liquids instead of water and then wonder why they don't feel well and can't maintain their health.

Here is a totally obvious, simple, and straightforward approach to taking care of one's health, the way Nature intended us to—that of simply supplying the living body with the appropriate water quality it must have for its very survival—but for some inexplicable reason it is not being utilized. People actually deprive themselves of something not only essential to life and health promoting but also so easily accessible. It is the irony of ironies. I guess the old adage that the simplest solutions in life are the ones most frequently overlooked is true.

OBTAINING ESSENTIAL NUTRIENTS FROM WATER AND DETOXING YOUR BODY

Obtaining essential nutrients from the water is a relatively recent discovery; it is believed to be vital to the future of our health. It is important, first, because water is a natural carrier and delivery system for nutrition. Second, it is important because many of the foods grown today are cultivated in agricultural areas that depend on the use of chemicals, so the foods have been depleted of valuable minerals and nutrients. Therefore, if your water of choice has been cleaned, purified properly of all contaminates and pollutants, and fortified and enhanced with a proper mineral and electrolyte additive, it becomes a superior carrier and advanced delivery system for mineral and electrolyte replacement, and for nutrition.

Providing the body with high-quality minerals and nutrition is important, but cleansing, balancing, and detoxifying the body of harmful acids and toxins is equally important. If there is in fact such a thing as a "secret" to health, cleansing of the inner body surely is it. The cleaner and more alive the water is to carry nutrition to the cell, the more active and able it will be to carry waste and toxins out of the cells and out of the body.

YOUR BODY PH AND THE IMPORTANCE OF MAINTAINING AN ALKALINE STATE

Like mineral and electrolyte balance the acid–alkaline balance of the body fluids plays a significant role in maintaining homeostasis and good health. The measure known as pH is the quantitative measure of the acidity or alkalinity of a substance or solution. The pH scale is based on the number of ions (positively charged atoms) in solution, and runs from 0 to 14. Ordinary water is measured as neutral—that is, it has a pH of 7.0. Numbers below 7.0 indicate an acid solution and those above 7.0 indicates a base or alkaline solution. Like salts, which are excellent conductors of electrical impulses in the human body, the inorganic compounds (compounds lacking carbon) known as acids and bases are electrolytes because they conduct electrical current once they have been ionized and dissolved in water.

The reason pH is so important for health is that the living cells are ultrasensitive to any changes in pH. Acid–base balance is therefore carefully maintained in the body fluids by the kidneys and lungs, and by certain chemicals called buffers. The acid–base balance, or pH, of blood is especially important because blood comes into close contact with nearly every living cell in the body. Blood pH is maintained within a very narrow range, from 7.35 to 7.45; a variance of more than a few tenths will most likely result in death. Acidic foods and beverages we consume affect the body's pH, as do environmental contaminants in the air we breathe and toxins that result from our agricultural practices. In fact the acid–alkaline state of our bodies and the need to maintain a healthy alkaline balance in our diets is a largely overlooked issue in health. The importance of drinking water with the correct pH and mineral content as well as consuming alkaline foods has become widely recognized by many in the health-aware community.

But not just any water is safe to drink. Next I will discuss the absolute tragedy of the public water system, better known as YOUR TAP WATER.

DON'T DRINK THE WATER UNLESS IT HAS BEEN PURIFIED

Research has shown that when body cells are properly hydrated, they become enlarged and trigger a healing mechanism. This healing mechanism is the result of such factors as a reduction of cellular acidity, increased fat burning, and repair of DNA. It has further been demonstrated that when the body becomes dehydrated, the cells become deflated and trigger the opposite of healing, or sickness, in the cells. This begins with a buildup of cellular acid and toxins, which leads to oxygen starvation and acceleration of the aging process.

Viewed from the perspective of one's health being significantly impacted by whether or not body cells are properly and sufficiently hydrated, we all need to be ever concerned about both the quality and quantity of the water we drink. As water beings on a water planet it is only logical for us to make this a high priority in our life. We have come a long way from the days of my childhood. When I was a kid, if you wanted a glass of water you simply went to the kitchen sink and drank your fill. Today, I'm sorry to say, much of the nation's groundwater and underground aquifers are contaminated with unhealthy levels of various chemicals.

Today, my attitude is, drink water but "Don't drink the *tap* water!" I don't care who says what about how pure or how clean commercial public "treated" tap water claims to be, I wouldn't drink tap water unless there was absolutely no choice. Many people drink tap water without so much as giving it a second thought. A host of chemicals, hazardous wastes, agricultural fertilizers, and industrial pollutants may also find their way into the water supply. All manner of other chemicals are deliberately added to the water supply at "purification" plants to counteract this and kill bacteria, and that water picks up metallic and plastic contaminants merely by flowing through the intricate web of pipelines, some of which are many decades old, before reaching you, and these metallic and plastic contaminants can contain an additional variety of such chemical pollutants.

RIGHT WATER FOR RIGHT HYDRATION

We are most fortunate to be living in an era when technological advances in water science have progressed to a staggering degree. Most people are not even remotely aware of the accomplishments that have been achieved in making available water that is infinitely superior to anything that was ever available in the past. Water is most definitely not "just water" any more. In only a few short decades we have progressed from the need to filter our basic tap water, to the need to seriously purify it, all the way to effectively enhancing our water to bring about maximum benefit.

I've heard people say, "Water is water—what difference does it make?" That simply is not accurate. In the same way that there is pure and clean air on the one hand and air that is polluted on the other; or food that is fresh and wholesome, and food that is overprocessed and unhealthy; there is water that is far superior to other water. In studying hydration, scientists have determined that water and hydration may be adequate around the outside of the cell, but without the right kind of water with the right electrical signature/mineral mix and proper surface tension, water flow into the cells is likely to be is impaired. The result is cellular dehydration.

Today, owing in large part to the advance of water science and technology there is a dizzying array of waters available on the market, including bottled waters—spring, artesian, filtered, mineral (carbonated and noncarbonated) purified/deionized, distilled, reverse osmosis, oxygenated, structured, micro-clustered, hexagonal, etc.—and home drinking water processors—distiller, reverse osmosis, activated carbon filter, softener, deionizer, mixed media, ionizer (electrolysis), vortexes—and combinations of these technologies.

With so many drinking water options on the market, the questions begging to be asked are:

"How do I choose the right water?"
"How do I know which water is best?"
"How can I be sure the water I'm drinking is what it is advertised to be?"
"How can I tell if my water meets the highest standards available?"

These are legitimate questions that anyone concerned with good health should be interested in having satisfactorily answered. They are most certainly the issues with which I personally want to be comfortable—especially in light of the fact that some bottled waters and water-treatment systems are going to be advertised and sold as superior when plainly they are not, but making this determination may be difficult for most consumers.

ABOUT BOTTLED WATER

That image of the clear mountain spring on the label may be misleading. Contrary to popular belief, bottled water isn't always cleaner and safer than tap water. According to the New York–based environmental advocacy group the National Resources Defense Council, about one third of the 100 brands of bottled water it tested violated stringent state and federal purity standards.[255] CNN reported that they had four bottled waters taken at random off the shelf and independently tested to see if they were everything they were advertised to be. Three out of four were not![256]

Like you, I struggle with these issues. I am deeply concerned about my health and I want to be certain that I am drinking only the very best water available anywhere—period! Knowing as I do the overwhelming importance of properly hydrating the cells of my body and the immeasurable good that results from doing so, I refuse to compromise even to the slightest degree when it comes to my drinking water. In the same way I know there are drinking water options that are not as good as they are advertised to be, I also know there have to be options that present the highest quality possible. I am always on the lookout for the most cutting-edge, up-to-date, uncompromising, finest water available.

THE SCIENCE OF WATER

I mentioned earlier that my decision to attach my name to a product is not something I do hastily. I am not a product-driven person—I won't endorse just anything for the sake of a check. Instead, I endorse and promote only a very select few; only ones that I am absolutely certain are of the highest quality and benefit for people who put their trust in me to lead them in the right direction. If I am not willing to consume a product myself, I would never recommend it to others, no matter what I was offered to do so.

In the mid 1980s when the first *Fit for Life* book was released I drank and highly recommended steam-distilled water. That was before many of the advances of water-science technology we know today had been made. I felt distilled was the best way to go at the time. Not that there is anything wrong with drinking distilled water—there isn't—but now I would recommend that it be remineralized with a small amount of ocean minerals, such as unprocessed sea salt. Distilled water remains infinitely superior to regular tap water; there's no comparison. But as knowledge has increased and advances have been made, superior water sources became available. At the close of the 1990s I recommended one of those that I found to be excellent; it has gone through some name changes but continues to be an outstanding water product. As time moves forward, more is learned and more is able to be achieved in water science; one must be on the alert all the time, and be flexible and ready to recognize a superior product when it comes along. I am always on "duty" and will continue to pass on to you anything I feel will help you in your efforts.

Today the water that has captured my attention and which I am convinced is an excellent and healthy drinking water for your family is the result of years of perfecting the purifying process.

This process starts out with an advanced water-treatment appliance based on the proven technologies of reverse osmosis and compressed coconut shell carbon. This provides a so-called "platform" of contaminant-free drinking water—and I do mean "contaminant-free." Virtually every category of water contaminant is reduced to insignificant levels with this consumer-friendly system. Here's a glance at what this technology duo is capable of removing from your drinking water:

Microbes. protozoan cysts, bacteria
Radioactivity. radium, radon
Inorganic contaminants. aluminum, antimony, arsenic, asbestos, barium, beryllium, cadmium, chromium, chloride, copper, cyanide, fluoride, lead, mercury, nickel, nitrate, nitrite, selenium, thallium
Synthetic organic contaminants (SOCs). insecticides, herbicides, pesticides, PCBs
Volatile organic contaminants (VOCs). benzene, petroleum products, plastics, solvents
Disinfectants. chlorine, chloramines, chlorine dioxide
Disinfection byproducts (DBPs). bromate, chlorite, halo acetic acids (HAAs), trihalomethanes (THMs)

Pharmaceutical endocrine disrupting chemicals and drugs. medicines, hormones, antibiotics, anti-depressants, illegal drugs, etc.

Personal care products. lotions, creams, cosmetics, cleaning products, etc.

Any other health writer would be ecstatic to be able to recommend such an effective product for removing the dizzying list of water contaminants. This process has taken the pursuit to a high level of consistent, clean and healthy water for you and your family.

Be that as it may, what I would ask of anyone reading this right now is not simply to take my word for what I'm saying, no matter how promising it may sound, but to do what I and many others have done—that is, to see for yourself. Think of the improvement in your health and life that is possible if what I've told you here is valid, sound, and true. Fortunately, the result of properly hydrating your body with extremely pure, high-quality water proves itself in a relatively short period of time.

Water is simply too important a factor in a person's health not to do whatever is necessary to seek out and consume the very finest available. Whether attempting to overcome ill-health or to maintain one's good health, properly hydrating the cells can only increase one's chances of success. Without a doubt, those desirous of experiencing the highest level of health available to them absolutely must pay as much attention to the quantity and quality of the water they drink as they do to the food they eat. Don't shortchange yourself when it comes to the water you drink and you will be glad for the remainder of your healthy and fit life.

To learn more about this exciting water system or to find out how to obtain it, you may call, toll-free, 877-335-1509, or go to the website, www.vpnutrition.com.

APPENDIX II

The Fountain of Youth?

You are probably familiar with the expression "Big things come in small packages." If that saying is true, then this little section certainly falls into that category. In only a few pages, you're going to learn about an astonishingly simple tool that, without exaggeration, will be one of the most profound and effective means by which you ensure for yourself that long, pain-free, and disease-free life that has been referred to throughout this book.

At public seminars I have given over the last twenty years or so, one question I always ask my audiences to respond to by raising their hands is, "How many people here love to eat?" Without fail, all in attendance throw their hands skyward as though they were reaching up to snatch hundred-dollar bills out of the air that have fallen from the ceiling. Many thrust both hands in the air with such enthusiasm you'd think I just asked them "How many people here would like a brand-new car of their choice, for free?" When the audiences were large, a thousand people or more, the upraised arms looked like a flock of flamingos coming in for a landing on the Serengeti Plain. After the fluttering and laughter subsided, I would explain what I have spoken of earlier: that each and every one of us will consume some 70 tons of food in our lifetime. So it certainly makes sense that if we're going to spend the amount of time necessary to obtain and eat 70 tons of food, we might just as well enjoy ourselves while we're doing it. Don't you agree?

FREEING THE DIGESTIVE SYSTEM REVISITED

I have already mentioned several times how much energy is required for the digestive process. The entire process of digestion and metabolism, the breaking down of the 70 tons of food, extraction and utilization of nutrients, and elimination of the wastes, will require more energy in your lifetime than all other uses of energy combined! Reflect on that for a while and you are sure to be impressed.

The digestion of food takes a huge amount of your energy, more than for anything else you do. Ever notice how tired you are after a meal? And the bigger the meal, the more tired you are. Remember last Thanksgiving? What did you do right after eating? As I asked earlier, did you look for your running shoes, or a couch? All over the world people have what is referred to as the "afternoon siesta." People eat and get tired because the digestive process demands the expenditure of such a high amount of energy.

You know, from the time you are born until the time you leave this life, you have a certain amount of life energy available to you. When it's gone, life is over. Since it is an unassailable, physiological fact that more of that energy will be used up for the digestive process than all other uses combined, does it not seem prudent beyond measure for you to make use of any possible means by which to either streamline the digestive process or in some manner reduce its burden? To me, the answer to that question is more obvious than the answer to the question: "Is the sun hot?" Reducing the burden of the digestive process can have but one long-term effect: It will improve the length and quality of your life. There's simply no doubt about that.

I have been studying and teaching a healthy lifestyle for over a quarter of a century now. All my books delineate methods you can use to decrease the work of the digestive process, to give it periodic rests; my ideas emphasize how important it is for you not to push the digestive process beyond its capabilities. I know many of you reading this right now have read *Fit for Life*, and that makes me extremely happy. And I know that there are those of you who have not read it. (We know who you are, incidentally.) *Fit for Life* contains an entire section on proper food combining, an approach that has many benefits. Food combining is a way to optimize energy from the digestive tract by not mixing protein (such as meat) with starches (such as potatoes or rice). The Number 1 benefit of the practice, as I explained earlier, is that it streamlines digestion. In this book, periodic monodieting shows you how to free a significant amount of energy from the digestive process which is, in turn, used by the body to thoroughly clean the lymph system; this ultimately prevents disease in the long term while dramatically improving all aspects of health in the short term.

Earlier, I shared with you the work of Dr. Roy Walford, who doubled the lifespan and dramatically improved the health of mice he experimented with merely by totally resting their digestive systems for two days a week. I also made the observation that animals in the wild or kept as pets will stop eating when they're sick or injured in order to free digestive energy for the healing process. And of course, children and adults also lose their appetites when they are "under the weather," which is, once again, the body's protective mechanism trying to divert to the healing process the energy that would be spent on digestion.

From what you have read so far, I'm certain that you see that anything you can do to reduce the work of your digestive system is an extremely wise thing to do. That being the case, I must say that I am astounded that one of the most simple, effective means by which anyone can immediately start to dramatically reduce the work of their digestive system, thereby ensuring a longer, healthier life, is largely unknown to the vast majority of the population. In fact, I wonder if there is anything, anywhere, that has the potential to do so much good that has been more overlooked and neglected. And what is this certain thing I am referring to? Enzymes!

LIFESAVING ENZYMES

To explain enzymes and what they do, I could launch into a convoluted, scientific dissertation about how amylase, which breaks down carbohydrates, splits starches into different disaccharides, or how pepsin, which works on proteins, splits proteins into smaller peptide chains, all so food can be broken down and made small enough to pass through the villi, the small pores of the intestines, and into the bloodstream. And if my goal was to cause you to skip this section, I would do just that. Instead, I wish to give you an ultrasimplified, totally nontechnical explanation, to be certain that you fully grasp and recognize the immense, lifesaving role enzymes play in your health. Anyone wishing a more detailed and scientific understanding of enzymes and their activity in the body can certainly read up on them.[257] But my primary goal here is to leave you with a newfound sense of the enormity of the role enzymes fulfill in our daily lives.

Enzymes are protein chemicals that carry an essential energy source needed for every chemical action and reaction that occurs in your body. We're talking about a number so immense you couldn't possibly comprehend it. Literally trillions upon trillions of chemical activities are taking place in your body right now. None would occur without enzymes. All life, plant or animal, requires enzymes to continue living. Enzymes *mean* life. Enzymes *are* life. Whenever you hear about or talk about your body doing something, anything, no matter what, that has anything whatsoever to do with the building, repairing, or maintaining of any part of your body, inside or out, enzymes are involved. And without them, nothing would get done. Life would cease to exist. The living body is under a great burden every day to produce the volume of enzymes necessary to run efficiently.

METABOLIC ENZYMES

There are three classes of enzymes you need to be aware of. First are metabolic enzymes, which are referred to as the body's labor force because virtually every activity of your body depends upon them. Without these power-packed little dynamos continually at work, you couldn't swallow, blink your eyes, circulate blood, breathe in and out, transform food into blood and muscle and bone, walk, talk, or anything else. The activities of the lymph system and its role in keeping you well while preventing pain and disease is entirely dependent, as is every other function of the body, on metabolic enzymes!

We all know how exceedingly important it is to eat a good diet so that the full complement of nutrients—the vitamins, minerals, essential fatty acids, and amino acids—can be made available to the body to carry out all of its functions. But no matter how pure the diet, no matter how many high-quality nutrients are introduced into the body, it all means nothing without metabolic enzymes.

I'll use a simple analogy to explain why this is so. If you wished to build a house, you could bring to the site all the materials you need to build it: lumber, hammers, nails, cement, bricks, mortar, insulation, wiring, roofing material, everything. But just putting all the materials on the site won't create the house. Unless the construction workers show up to assemble all the materials, the house will not be built. No matter how plentiful the materials, no matter how high the quality of the materials, if there are no construction workers, there is no house. Metabolic enzymes are your body's "construction workers." Without them, nothing gets done, and I mean nothing.

Here is the single most important fact about metabolic enzymes that you must be aware of. There is a finite number of metabolic enzymes that can be produced by your body. I want to be absolutely certain you know exactly what I'm saying. Your body can produce a certain number of metabolic enzymes, and no more! You can, you *will*, run out of them! And there is a word to describe what takes place when you run out of them. It's called death. That's what dying means. There are no more metabolic enzymes to carry out the functions of life, so life ends. It would be as though when you were born, you were given a bank account that contained a certain amount of money for your entire lifetime from which you could remove, but not add, money. You can either be prudent with that money and make it last a long time, or you can squander it and let it run out sooner than you wish. So it is with metabolic enzymes. It's an extremely simple equation. The more metabolic enzymes you require and use up, the unhealthier you will be and the shorter your life will be. The fewer metabolic enzymes you require and use up, the healthier you will be and the longer you will live. And of that, there is simply no doubt. Anything, and I mean anything you can do to use up fewer of your metabolic enzymes is obviously one of the most intelligent and life-enhancing practices you can cultivate as regards your health and longevity.

DIGESTIVE ENZYMES AND FOOD ENZYMES

The second type of enzymes are digestive enzymes. The function of these enzymes should be fairly obvious. That's right, they are involved in the specific job of digestion. Food in the stomach is a Number 1 priority for the human body, and digestive enzymes are required to perform the process of digestion of food in the stomach. Pretty simple stuff.

Now, right here I would like to jump to food enzymes, which are the third type of enzyme, as a discussion will clarify the role of digestive enzymes. All food that has grown out of the ground, as part of God's grand scheme of things, has contained in it all the necessary enzymes to break it down in the body for digestion. Before going into the immense importance of food enzymes, I need to give you some corollary information that will help you more fully appreciate the importance and significance of not only food enzymes but also digestive and metabolic enzymes.

There are many elements that set humans apart from all other animal species on the planet. One of the more impressive differences is our more highly developed brain and our ability to think and reason. It is what allows us to accomplish so much of what is not even in the realm of possibility for all the other so-called lower animals. Ironically, it also is what gets us into trouble as regards our health and well-being, trouble that the lower animals don't have to contend with, trouble that is associated with diet, nutrition, and health. For example, do you realize that we humans are the only species on earth to cook our foods before we eat them? We are also, not coincidentally, the only species to suffer from the diseases of affluence discussed earlier, which are heart disease, cancer, diabetes, osteoporosis, and obesity. Food keeps us alive; that is a simple, self-evident fact. Stop eating and you die. But way back in history, we started cooking the life out of our foods before eating them and we have been paying the price with ill health and premature death ever since.

Animals in nature do not ever eat cooked food and they do not suffer from the diseases of affluence. There are, of course, exceptions to this, but those exceptions come into play only as other animal species come into close contact with humans. And the closer the contact, the more disease occurs. For example, animals in zoos or animals we take as pets, or animals that are in some way forced to interact with humans, suffer from the same diseases of affluence that afflict humans. Because we feed them our cooked food! Could anything on earth be more obvious?

I must share with you one phenomenally impressive study that is recognized the world over as one of the most convincing studies on this subject ever conducted. I lived in Los Angeles for thirty-five years, so I did the bulk of my research at the UCLA Medical Library, one of the best in the country. I spent hundreds of hours there poring over studies to substantiate much of my work. Finding this amazing study, which I wrote about in *Fit for Life II*, was like winning the lottery. The study has come to be known as Pottenger's Cats.[258]

Dr. Francis Pottenger carried out a meticulous, thorough, ten-year experiment using 900 cats placed on controlled diets. Only two items of food were used and were given either in their raw or cooked state. The results were so overwhelmingly conclusive and convincing that there can be no doubt whatsoever of living, uncooked food's superiority over cooked food. The cats fed only the living, raw food produced healthy kittens year after year. There was no ill health, no disease, and no premature death. Death came to those cats only as the natural consequence of old age. However, the cats fed on the same food, cooked, developed every one of humanity's modern ailments— heart disease, cancer, kidney and thyroid disease, pneumonia, paralysis, loss of teeth, arthritis, difficulty in labor, diminished sexual interest, diarrhea, irritability so intense that the cats were dangerous to handle, liver impairment, and osteoporosis. The excrement from these cats was so toxic that weeds refused to grow in the soil fertilized with it, whereas weeds proliferated in the stools from the cats fed the living, uncooked food. Here is the clincher: The first generation of kittens born to the group of cats who were fed only cooked food were sick and abnormal. The second generation were often born diseased or dead. By the third generation the mothers were sterile. Dr. Pottenger conducted similar tests on white mice and the results coincided exactly with those of the tests run on cats.

So what do Pottenger's Cats and cooked food have to do with my discussion of enzymes? Just this: Far less heat than is required to cook food entirely obliterates all food enzymes. I want to be certain that you are clear on what I am saying. When you cook your food, the enzymes necessary to break down that food in your body are destroyed. Not some of them. All of them. And they're not merely degraded or made to be less effective. They are, every last one, completely and totally wiped out. This sets up quite a predicament for your body. One that has some very negative results. You see, food in the stomach, as I said, is a Number 1 priority for your body. Food can't simply sit around in your stomach; it has to be dealt with immediately. But if the food has been cooked, the enzymes that would have done that job are gone. At this crucial moment, the wisdom and intelligence of the body snaps into action and calls upon the mechanism in the body that produces metabolic enzymes and forces it to produce the digestive enzymes necessary to digest the food. Now remember, this mechanism that produces metabolic enzymes is the very same one that determines the length and quality of your life. We know that this mechanism can only produce a certain number of enzymes, and then life ends. So every time you eat something that is cooked, you are literally inviting ill health and shortening your life.

The reason this is so is that when you suddenly force the metabolic enzyme mechanism to produce digestive enzymes, the work that the metabolic enzymes would have been doing to keep everything working efficiently and effectively, thereby keeping you well and healthy, is compromised and thwarted. The very mechanism in the body designed to keep you healthy and energetic is kept from doing its job. If your lymph system is overburdened, that means your body is working to decrease the amount of waste that has accumulated, which can ultimately make you sick. Every time you eat cooked food, you not only lessen the effectiveness of your body's labor force (metabolic enzymes) that is trying to cleanse and strengthen your body, but you also rob unnecessarily from the very mechanism that determines how long and how well you will live. And that has to be the last thing on earth you would ever want to intentionally do.

ENZYMES

Right about now you might be thinking that I'm getting around to convincing you to become a total raw fooder, eating only uncooked food. Nope! That is not my intention. Hey, I like cooked food and I'm not about to give it up. So I'm sure as heaven not going to suggest that you do. Now, without question, the amount of uncooked food I eat does far outweigh the cooked food I consume, but no, I'm not going to suggest that we stop eating all cooked food. But here is what I *am* going to suggest, and it is the very purpose of these few pages.

Thanks to technological advances that did not exist when I wrote *Fit for Life*, there are now available to one and all what are called live plant enzymes, which can be taken just prior to eating anything cooked, that do the job that the cooked-away enzymes were supposed to do. They, in effect, put the life that was cooked out of your food back in so you can live on it. They come in very small capsules, they are totally nontoxic, they have no side effects other than increased health and longevity, and they prevent the unnecessary squandering of your precious metabolic-enzyme capacity. These pharmaceutical-grade, live plant enzymes are grown and harvested in a laboratory setting without compromising them with heat. In my opinion, the ability to make these live plant enzymes available to us is one of the most significant and beneficial advances of the twentieth century. If there is a substance that could rightly be called the fountain of youth, this is surely it.

From the day I found out these live plant enzymes were available, until now, I have been taking them whenever I eat anything cooked. No matter where I am, no matter who I'm with, no matter what I'm doing, I always carry them with me and take them before eating any cooked food. At this point in my life, I would just as soon pass on eating than to eat something cooked without my enzymes. I'm serious. I simply don't eat anything cooked if I don't have my enzymes with me, and as much as I love to eat, you can be sure that if you run into me somewhere, I'll have capsules with me. If I don't, then you can be just as sure that I'm not on my way to a restaurant, unless, of course, I plan on eating salad or something else that has not been cooked.

I did some research into which enzymes were the absolute finest, purest, most high-quality live plant enzymes available anywhere in the world, and those are the only ones I take. Consider the words of Dr. Edward Howell, the man considered to be the father of enzyme nutrition:

> I like to think of life as an integration of enzyme reactions. Life ends when the worn out metabolic enzyme activity of the body machine drops to such a low point that it is unable to carry on vital enzyme reactions. This is the true trademark of old age. Old age and debilitated metabolic enzyme activity are synonymous. If we post-

pone the debilitation of metabolic enzyme activity, what we now call old age could become the glorious prime of life.[259]

Allow me to ask you a question. Would there by any possibility at all, *any,* of you going to the bank on a regular basis, taking out your hard-earned cash, and then using it as toilet paper? Any chance at all? Can you even think of anything that would be more absurd and ridiculous? No? Well, I can. I can think of one thing more preposterous than using your cash as toilet paper and that would be using up the metabolic enzymes in your body that keep you healthy and alive, in order to digest cooked food that you could have taken live plant enzymes for. If a long life free of pain, ill health, and disease is one of the goals you have for yourself and your loved ones, then start using live plant enzymes *now!* Many people who have started using these digestive enzymes upon my recommendation, have reported to me that the bloated feeling they customarily experience after a meal has completely disappeared since the regular use of these enzymes. Others have told me that other digestive disorders that usually require some kind of digestive aid to quell the discomfort (gas, pain, heartburn, acid indigestion) have also disappeared. Do this for yourself—you're worth it.

For information on how to obtain the live plant enzymes I use called DiamondZyme, call VP Nutrition, toll free, 877-335-1509. You may also view the information on their website at www.vpnutrition.com.

In the future, the need to take live plant enzymes with cooked food will be as well established as today's dictum that to acquire and maintain a high level of health we must exercise and eat right. Don't wait! Take advantage of this information now and get a jump on it. You will be glad for the rest of your *long and healthy* life.

APPENDIX III

Edutrition® and Supplements

As I stated earlier my goal through the pages of this book is to educate you about nutrition and nutritional supplements, and how this information can empower you to make choices that will improve your health. I know the subject of supplements is of great importance for many of you. In this section I wish to supply you with the most cutting-edge information on the subject. To that end the next several pages will discuss the subject of Edutrition®.

Many of the references that I make in this section which will be updated regularly on the website www.vpnutri tion.com. As more and more research unfolds, I hope to keep you informed through the pages of this site, as well as with a free monthly e-newsletter. Be sure to call 877-335-1509, 941-966-9727, or e-mail info@vpnutrition.com, and you will automatically be added to the free newsletter list. Please pay special attention to the next few pages, as you are about to get a real eye-opening Edutrition®.

DEVASTATED FOOD = DEVASTATED HEALTH

The magnificent human body has been designed to be nourished simply by eating food. But nowadays, finding food "worth eating" has become a complex task, as the quality of our food spirals lower with each passing year. Look at the following reports:

UK and U.S. government statistics indicate that levels of trace minerals in fruit and vegetables fell by up to 76 percent between 1940 and 1991. (So, mathematically, you eat one apple and get the nutritional value of less than a quarter of an apple!)

In contrast there is growing evidence that organic fruit and vegetables generally contain more nutrients than nonorganic food. The Soil Association conducted a systematic review of the evidence comparing the vitamin and mineral content of organic and conventionally grown food. An independent review of the evidence found that organic crops had significantly higher levels of all 21 nutrients analyzed compared with conventional produce—the levels ranged from 14 to 27 percent higher. That brings organic food to the level of conventional food in the 1970s, or around 50 percent—so with organic food you now have about half an apple. The question is can you be healthy eating food reduced in nutritional value by 50–76 percent?

Then there is the issue of enzymes, which are used in every function of the living body. You have to understand that digestive enzymes are different from liver enzymes or brain enzymes or heart enzymes. The blood itself has different enzymes. The types of enzymes that work inside the cell are different in their functions from the ones working outside of the cell. Sad to say, the majority of us, whether apparently ill or not, have one or more blocked enzyme systems due to the toxic environment we live in. These systems need to be unblocked before we can derive any lasting benefit from nutrients.

WHAT DOES ALL THIS MEAN?
THE BIG PICTURE

What does all this mean? The food we eat, whether conventional or organic, is depleted by 50 to 76 percent of what it was meant to be. The majority of our food is genetically altered, overprocessed, and loaded with pesticides and other chemicals and toxins. This assault on our system translates into exactly what we don't want: rapid aging, feeling tired, blocked enzyme systems, all kinds of deficiency symptoms, and greater risk of disease. Supplying the body with high levels of nutrients can mean feeling great; low levels can mean feeling lifeless. Deficient nutrient levels also mean being at risk for the dreaded chronic diseases that have become so prevalent today: arthritis, prostatitis, diabetes, asthma, autism spectrum disorders, heart disease, and cancer.

To get protection from the effects of toxic damage and stress, it is obvious that regular food isn't the whole answer. It's a challenge to get sufficient amounts of nutrients from food, including food that is "organically grown." To fill the void many have turned to nutritional supplements. The question remains how do you go about determining which supplements to choose?

Natural vitamins taken from once-living whole foods is the best choice for use in our bodies. Whole-food ingredients will be easily absorbed by the body. They are made from pure raw materials that naturally contain the hundreds of "co-factors" (other nutrients the body needs to absorb vitamins). When co-factors are missing, as they are in synthetic vitamins, the body may treat the vitamin as a foreign substance and eliminate it or pass it whole, or it may even grab the needed co-factors from its own organs, bones, muscles, or other tissue. In other words, your body starts eating itself! Over time, this depletes the body, causing disease and degeneration.

Clearly choosing natural whole-food vitamins is in your own best interests, but where to look, whom to trust? In the next few pages, I will recommend a company and nutritional supplements that I personally use. I believe these will be as helpful in your search for vibrant health as they have been for me. This company VP Nutrition can be contacted by calling 877-335-1509 or visiting their website, www.vpnutrition.com.

SUPPLEMENTS

Taken as a complementary protocol these four products are beneficial for anyone—with health issues or none at all. For those in apparently good health, this protocol can be a wonderful preventative, assisting your body in "maintaining a clean house." For more information on these homeopathic products, please see www.fitforlifetime.com/links.php; or you may purchase them on the Web, at www.vpnutrition.com, or call toll free 877-335-1509

LifeGreens Powder—Natural Multivitamin Supplement with the Antioxidant Power of 25+ Servings of Vegetables and Fruit

LifeGreens contains a full range of amino acids plus essential vitamins and minerals. LifeGreens Powder tastes great and can be mixed in smoothies, is a phytonutrient powder mix loaded with certified organic, whole food plant extracts. It's a super blend of completely natural vitamin, ionic trace mineral, enzymes, antioxidants, phytonutrients and symbiotic intestinal flora for energy, metabolism, digestion, detoxification, revitalization and longevity support.

DiamondZyme—Digestive Enzyme

DiamondZyme enhances the digestion and assimilation of food and supplements while reducing the body's need to produce digestive enzymes. Over the course of many years, we use up much of our enzyme potential, which is necessary for proper food digestion. When this happens, our ability to keep up with our bodies' digestive enzyme requirements begins to suffer. This deficiency may lead to malabsorption and poor nutrition along with digestive problems. Supplementing with a high-potency plant-based enzyme formula may aid in preventing this process. It is usually best to take 6 capsules a day. If you eat 4–6 times a day, take one at each meal. If you eat 3 times a day, take 2 at a time.

DiamondZyme is primarily recognized as a maintenance formulation for those who have addressed their imbalances and now have a need to maintain that balance, or for those who suffer from minor or occasional digestive problems. It is ideal for children or anyone who has difficulty swallowing capsules. The DiamondZyme capsule is among the smallest available.

DiamondZyme Plus—Extra Strength Live Plant Enzymes

DiamondZyme Plus represents VP's most potent digestive enzyme formula. It has been designed to support the digestion of proteins, fats, carbohydrates, and fiber. DiamondZyme Plus is more potent than DiamondZyme. It contains four more enzymes and is approximately three times stronger than DiamondZyme in most categories.

DiamondZyme Plus has been formulated to address the more serious issues some people have to deal with. It will do everything DiamondZyme does and more. Since the formula is more potent and contains several more enzymes, fewer capsules are required. One capsule per meal is usually sufficient to address even the most serious digestive issue. DiamondZyme Plus is also ideal for anyone suffering from health issues not necessarily associated with digestion. When stress is reduced to the system responsible for breaking down and assimilating the foods consumed, then more energy and thus more metabolic enzymes are made available to other systems of the body responsible for overall health.

RenewZyme

RenewZyme, which is formulated to speed recovery and repair tissue, contains the highest amount of proteolytic enzymes (enzymes that break down proteins) that have exhibited anti-inflammatory qualities. After an injury some capillaries may be damaged, making them incapable of carrying fluid to and from the damaged tissue. The result is pain, swelling, redness, heat, and loss of function. By repairing the capillaries, bruises, swelling, and pain may be reduced. The enzymes in RenewZyme have been shown to improve circulation and speed recovery. Once in the bloodstream proteolytic enzymes enhance blood flow. Additionally, these same proteases have been known to support the immune system and have antioxidant qualities.

Some of VP Nutrition's Other Products

VP Nutrition works hard to provide quality enzyme and nutritional supplements
Some of their other products include:

Life Coral: Complete marine coral calcium supplement supports bone and pH balance.
Life Magnesium: Supports over 300 enzyme-related processes including cardiac, muscle, and nerve function, and the production of ATP for energy. Especially helpful for ASDs. Features highly absorbable magnesium lysinate, glycinate chelate and the patented di-magnesium malate from Albion Laboratories..
Life D3: Natural form of D3 in a micellized (water-soluble) form, offers special support for immune, bone, neurological health.

Life EFA: A balanced blend of Essential Fatty Acids from flax, borage, and fish oil; supports cardiovascular, nervous, and immune systems and is helpful for ASDs.

Life Max B: This B complex supplement helps support brain, liver, and nerve function.

Life Immuno PRP Spray: Supports proper regulation of the thymus gland and cytokine balance.

To see these and more products visit them on the Web at www.vpnutrition.com.

Contact Page

For more information on the educational organizations or products I have mentioned in this book please call toll free 877-335-1509. Outside the U.S. call 941-966-9727, or go to www. vpnutrition.com.

To Purchase Products

You may purchase all the products I have mentioned and much more by contacting:

VP NUTRITION
P.O. Box 811
Osprey, FL 34229
877-335-1509 or 941-966-9727
www.vpnutrition.com

NOTES TO THE APPENDICES

255. "Bottled Water Watch," *New Age Magazine,* July/August 1999.
256. Ibid.
257. Howell, Edward, M.D., *Enzyme Nutrition,* Avery, NJ, 1985; Lopez, D.A., M.D., Williams, R.M., M.D., Miehlke, K., M.D., *Enzymes: The Fountain of Life,* Neville Press, SC, 1994.
258. Pottenger, Francis M., "The Effect of Heat Processed Foods and Metabolized Vitamin D Milk on the Dento-Facial Structures of Experimental Animals," *American Journal of Orthodontics & Oral Surgery,* No. 8, Aug. 1946.
259. Howell, Edward, M.D., *Enzyme Nutrition,* Avery, NJ, 1985; Lopez, D.A., M.D., Williams, R.M., M.D., Miehlke, K., M.D., *Enzymes: The Fountain of Life,* Neville Press, SC, 1994.

INDEX

One of Harvey's lifelong concerns was making sure people have enough to eat. His longtime friend Tony Robbins continues this important work through his efforts with the group Feeding America. In support of that mission we continue to inform people about how to be involved and support this critical project. Visit feedingamerica.org/1billionmeals.

Tony Robbins has dedicated his life to giving to others. From initiating programs in over 1,500 schools and providing fresh water to 100,000 people a day in India to ensuring nuns in San Francisco have a place to operate their soup kitchen, Tony's actions demonstrate his belief that when we give more, we become more.

You may have heard Tony talk about one of his recent philanthropic projects, Feeding America. If you're interested in joining him on his mission to end hunger, donate to this organization via the links below. Take action today!

HELP TONY SUPPORT THESE EFFORTS:

FEEDING AMERICA *and its*

1 Billion Meals Challenge

Tony's goal? Providing 1 BILLION MEALS by 2025.

The 1 Billion Meals Challenge aims to provide 100 million meals per year through 2025 to families struggling with hunger in the United States. In the last five years, Tony has helped provide more than 517 million meals to people in need through the Feeding America network of 200 food banks. Tony has committed a lead gift to support Feeding America and the 1 Billion Meals Challenge. Help match this gift to double the impact for kids and families in need.

Join Tony in his 1 Billion Meals Challenge with Feeding America today! Visit feedingamerica.org/1billionmeals.